I0472329

PSYCHOTHERAPY
FROM THE PATIENT'S PERSPECTIVE

LET'S GET BETTER BOOK SERIES II

HAMILTON PEIRSOL, PSY. D., L.P.C., C.A.P., CAADC, M.B.A.
©2019
SAVANNAH, GEORGIA

AMAZON PRESS

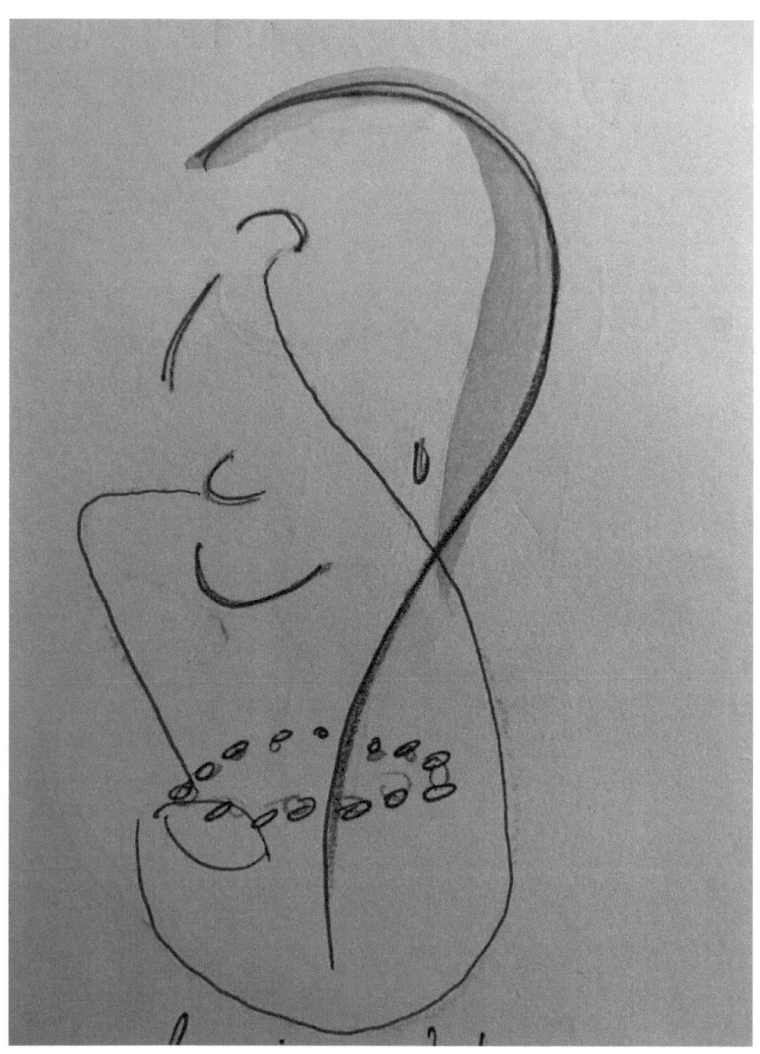

REFLECTIONS

Retitled watercolor on paper canvas with sketch tones
©2019 Dr. Peirsol

OUTLINE

PSYCHOTHERAPY
FROM THE PATIENT'S PERSPECTIVE

INTRODUCTION

That first time I stepped into a therapist's office I was nervous. I did not know what to expect. I knew there was something wrong, but I didn't know what. I was a college freshman and was struggling to find my way in the world. Thought I wanted to go to seminary to be a priest but soon realized after meeting my psychotherapist that there was something different.

Anytime someone comes into therapy, I always try to remember that first day myself, the awkwardness of it all and that pure thick fog of just not knowing what will happen gripping you, not knowing what to say much less how to sit or what to do other than to be there and try to speak. I am sure I fumbled with my words then, was as fragile as a butterfly's feather on its wing and was clueless as to what the therapist must have been seeing in me that first day.

This book is intended to help prepare you for your psychotherapy experience, to assist you in the art of the experience itself, what to expect and how to make the most of it.

In **Chapter 1**, *A Broader Perspective for Therapy*, I have attempted to provide information from the literature, to provide some of the minimum expectations one might anticipate from a therapist when they come into psychotherapy. It reviews what is vitally important to ensure the psychotherapy works effectively. It starts with the importance of the therapeutic alliance and what that actually is and continues by elaborating upon some of the characteristics of a good therapeutic relationship, and what one can expect from their therapist once they are in the therapeutic arena. There are *10-Therapy Factors* to consider when entering and following through with one's therapy experience, each being highlighted in practical ways for you as the reader anticipating the start of your psychotherapy experience.

Chapter 2, *Case Studies of Psychotherapy*, highlights the nuts and bolts of what actual patients feel is important for them in psychotherapy, what they experienced and what they gained from attending psychotherapy themselves. I present psychotherapy from several patient's points of view, talking about their feelings and fears coming in and what they learned to do to get the most out of it. They share their takeaway and what they would advise for the next person entering psychotherapy. Some of them tell you more details than others, what their dealing with and what they are going through. Ultimately, the intention was for these particular patients to feel like they were able to give back as a way of deeper healing for them in helping others similarly to feel better, too. As a result of their sharing their stories anonymously, they will always know there are others out there better off for what they went through, able to learn from their experience so maybe they don't have to go through what they did the way they did when they did.

These are real patients with true stories. Their identity is altered so no one can be recognized. The case studies consist of the patients answering seven (7) different clusters of questions. The questions they draw from are listed in the following next few paragraphs.

What are case studies and what is the benefit of looking at them? A case study in this context is a review of specific elements of an individual's personal experience of psychotherapy as well as my observations of the patient during that experience. It considers what they perceive, feel and think and draws conclusions as a result of all the case studies put together. Each case is different but there might be similar factors not evident, and by reviewing each case individually, these unique qualities will have a chance to be highlighted. Such highlights will stem from the following questions asked of each patient as they reflect on their psychotherapy experience:

1. What triggered your awareness that you should seek psychotherapy or the need to see a counselor in the first place? Go into as much detail as you like. What were your initial impressions of needing to see someone, what were the issues you were having to address, what did you think of psychotherapy then before you even went, and what were you feeling about it before you even got started?

2. What was it like for you at first, realizing that this is what you need to do, having to find a therapist you liked, your first experience of going to the office, checking in and having that first meeting? Looking back, what was that first session like for you? From your point of view, what was it like being a patient or client in psychotherapy? What was your takeaway and what do you wish you had known then that you know now prior to that first meeting?

3. What made you decide to go back after the first session? What came of the initial stages of your treatment/therapy and what do you recall most about your experience early on? Looking back is there anything you wish

you would have known or done differently now looking back on that initial period?

4. What did you discover along the way, things about yourself that you might not have expected, things you liked and things you didn't? What do you remember most about the most difficult part(s) of the therapy experience? Looking back, what were some of the initial changes you started to make as a result of the therapy? How did your point of view of psychotherapy start to change during this process and what do you think of it now looking back?

5. What made the therapy work for you? What did you learn most about yourself that was a surprise and what changed for you, in life, your relationships, etc. in the process of being a patient or client in psychotherapy? Looking back was there anything about yourself you discovered that you wished you had known before going to therapy and what difference do you think that may have made in your life if you had known it prior to therapy?

6. Looking back on your therapy experience, thinking about others that could have learned from what you experienced as a result of therapy, what is there you would want to tell them if you could that maybe as

a result of what you learned they would be able to avoid the difficulties you experienced? What is it that you would want to tell them about psychotherapy that you wished you knew before now so that maybe they too could get the most out of it if they chose to go?

7. What are the most important things you have learned as a result of your experience in psychotherapy? What do want to be sure others know from your point of view about your experience in psychotherapy, what you want to give back if you had the chance to tell them now?

Each patient takes the time to reflect on these questions and has written out their own responses. I have reviewed each case description provided with the patient and discussed together what would be printed. Each of the cases presented are their stories in their own words from their actual point of view about their experience with psychotherapy.

In **Chapter 3**, *Finding Your Way in Therapy*, I have attempted to assess the combination of all the case studies, their responses, and have provided a summary of what some of the primary vantage points appear to be as takeaways for you the reader toward having a better experience in psychotherapy from the patients' perspective. As a result, I have provided the following *7-Points of View* broken down by each of set of questions:

1) What are the general first impressions of the idea of going to psychotherapy?
2) What is that first session really like?
3) What can you expect getting started?
4) What might be an unexpected part of it?
5) What will you discover as result of psychotherapy?
6) What is the ultimate takeaway from attending psychotherapy?
7) What's the best advice one can offer as a result of attending psychotherapy themselves?

These *Seven (7)-Points of View from the Patient's Perspective* range from what it was like prior to coming, to having that first session, what to expect and what to anticipate. As a result of reviewing each case study, I have been able to determine approximately *12-Takeways from Psychotherapy* to offer others and *4-Rules of Thumb for Psychotherapy* to follow as a way of getting the most out of one's experience with psychotherapy, as well as *Seven Promises of Psychotherapy Working* to verify its value.

In the final chapter, Chapter 4, *Clinical Guidelines of Therapy,* I attempt to provide specific practical suggestions that will improve one's clinical experience in psychotherapy. In effect, after looking over the case studies, combined with twenty-five plus years of experience working with clients, I highlight ways that a newcomer or even seasoned patient can get more from their psychotherapy experience, all from the feedback from patients over the years of practicing.

In conclusion, I summarize that psychotherapy can be a welcomed addition to one's life experience, it can instill hope and curiosity to life, as well as provide results one might be looking for in improving one's life; that it is life altering and that one will benefit the sooner they can get started. I close with acknowledgments and the list of references utilized to help put the material together for *Psychotherapy: From the Patient's Perspective.*

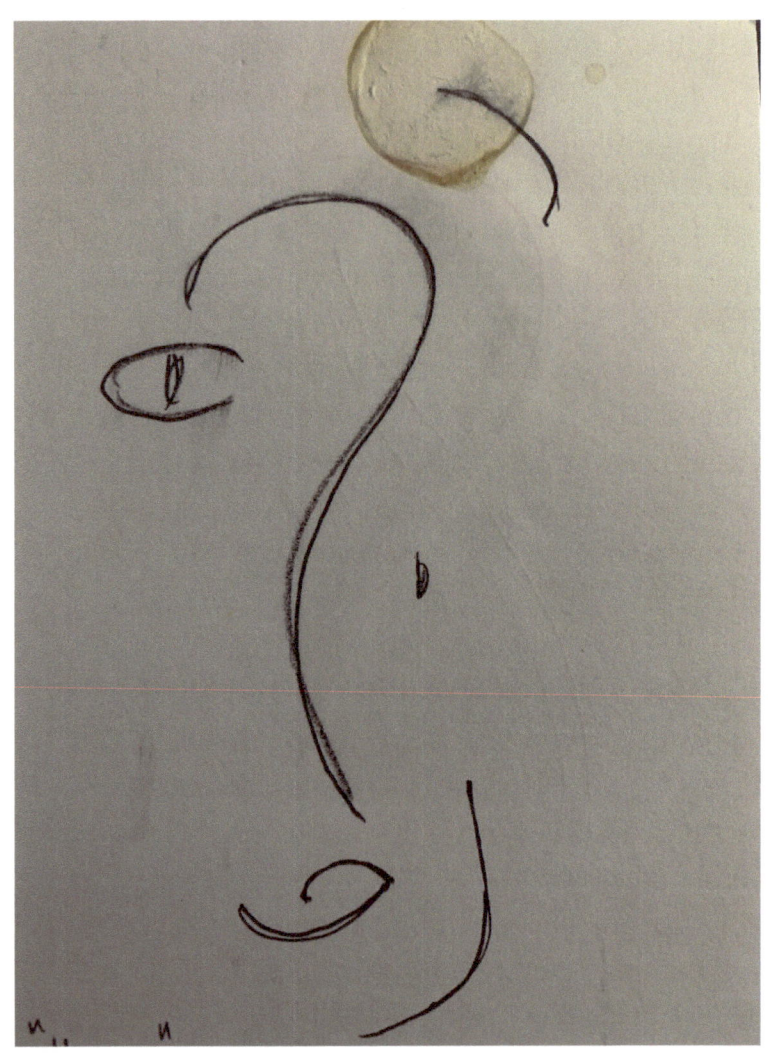

Perspective.

Watercolor on paper canvas with sketch tones
©2019 Dr. Peirsol

CHAPTER 1
A BROADER PERSPECTIVE FOR THERAPY

Before we get steeped in the case studies, let me review some of the literature, what the research has to say about what patients might be looking for in psychotherapy, especially from the therapeutic relationship. It is important coming into therapy that one be prepared to know what they should be receiving, what is most beneficial for you as the consumer of psychotherapy.

One of the mainstays of psychotherapy is the alliance established between patient and therapist. There is a strong connection in the literature between what is called the therapeutic alliance and the outcome of psychotherapy. This so-called alliance is the actual relationship between therapist and client, the dynamics and the innerworkings that go on in the relationship. One of the reasons for its importance is because so much is dependent upon how well the two inter-relate with one another throughout the therapeutic experience. Another reason is that some would consider the alliance itself as a healing agent for the therapy. Think of it as having a close ally to rely upon in times of trouble, a confidant to who one can turn for support. Similarly, the therapeutic relationship is built upon such confidence that a great deal of energy is put forth to ensure the alliance is a strong for client and therapist alike.

According to Hersoug et al. (2001), there are very specific factors however that a patient may be looking for in the alliance with a therapist. This will be important to review because it will help you as the reader facilitate what is important to you as you consider psychotherapy for yourself or a loved one, in addition to the insights we intend to gain from the various case studies to follow. There are three (3) factors Hersoug and her colleagues speak of that appear to be important to patients while in therapy and they are as follows: 1) the importance of "less self-directed hostility" 2) "more perceived social support," and 3) a "higher degree of comfort with closeness in interpersonal relationships." [i]

One certainly can appreciate the value of having a relationship with a therapist where there is less hostility associated with the experience. It is a matter of how the therapist treats the client, as cold and aloof, or warm and friendly. Naturally, most people would respond more favorably to the kinder mindset and so it is only natural this might be one of the valued characteristics to be found in one's therapist.

The value of experiencing social support is also quite noticeably important as well for anyone going through a somewhat challenging situation as is usually the case in psychotherapy. If the therapist can provide greater support socially, in an emotionally and personally supportive way, all the better to ensure a better therapy alliance, improving in the long run a better outcome of the therapy.

Moreover, the better able the therapist can relate socially especially in dealing with the "closeness" of the therapeutic alliance then the better the outcome of the therapy as well. Lingiardi et al. (2018) state "therapists' interpersonal functioning and skills showed the strongest evidence of a direct effect on treatment outcomes." [ii] Being able to handle the ebbs and flows of interpersonal relationships, having fine tuned interpersonal skills, can make a great deal of difference for certain patients adjusting more effectively to the changes they need to acquire as a result of therapy.

In addition, according to Nissen-Lie et al. (2015), it is apparent that patients similarly are averse to negative reactions displayed by the therapist in-session and are sensitive to the levels of anxiety shown by therapist during any therapy.[iii] This would suggest a heightened level of sensitivity certainly on the patients part during any therapeutic endeavor, interestingly tuned-in to the negative displays of behavior by therapists especially. And, it seems somewhat natural, a patient might be averse to the anxiety displayed by a therapist especially given that patients are tending to deal with enough anxiety themselves much less having to deal that of their therapist.

Patients tend to be very aware also of whether or not a therapist is engaged with them or not. They can experience "the effects of the therapist's disengaged feelings (i.e., bored, tired of, sleepy, indifferent, aloof)" and this can significantly contribute to a negative outcome in the therapy. What is suggested for the patient if the therapist is disengaged is to engage the therapist about how disengaged they appear to be. It is important to "discuss the patient-therapist interaction." [iv]

Also, patients are influenced a great deal by the way a therapist emotionally responds or not in therapy. From the patient's perspective this is important also to know because the therapist's emotional responsiveness can influence the level of awareness a therapist will have of a patient's personality or not. The outcome of the therapy is similarly affected by these levels of emotional responsiveness. Moreover, their emotional responses can equally "influence patient resistance and elaboration, mediate the influence of the therapist's interventions and influence (the) therapeutic alliance." [v] So, it is vital for the client/patient to openly discuss with the therapist their emotional reactions to the therapeutic experience. This can occur simply by the client/patient asking the therapist to elaborate on any of their reactions during the session. This type of dialogue will help further facilitate a patient sharing more or less and improve the likelihood of a therapist's intervention when trying to help.

Continuing further with the value of the patient's perspective of the therapist, it is also important to keep in mind that patients may be looking for multiple ways to further the relationship with the therapist toward a good outcome. What will help however is if the therapist has certain "personal attributes such as being flexible, honest, respectful, trustworthy, confident, warm, interested, and open." These characteristics were especially important and "found to contribute positively to the alliance." Moreover, the ability for the therapist to disperse certain techniques is also important. It is recognized that a therapist ability in "exploration, reflection, noting past therapy success, (having) accurate interpretation, facilitating the expression of affect, and attending to the patient's experience" are all vital to improving the alliance as well and subsequently the therapeutic outcomes.[vi]

Other literature cites the importance of how a therapist can attach more specifically to a patient and their mannerisms. In fact, how a therapist attaches emotionally or not is more of a contributing factor to the therapeutic alliance than is necessarily the therapeutic approach or orientation of the therapist. What this suggests for the patient is the importance of engaging as much as is possible with their therapist in an effort to establish as a close a relationship as is possible. The more available the therapist then the higher the likelihood a better attachment between the two. In fact, the specific style of "securely attaching" by the therapist then the better the relationship will be. What this suggests is that from a patient's perspective, the therapist needs to be secure in their way of engaging and interacting, connecting confidently and interacting positively with the patient for the outcome to be more viable as a result of a stronger alliance. Conversely, if the attachment style of therapist is in any way an "anxious" type of attachment, then the therapy is likely to derail due to a poorer alliance being established. [vii] [viii]

Furthermore, patients need to have a therapist who is able to relate to them and their relational style rather than vice versa. The more aware a patient can be of the relational ability of a therapist to understand them as a patient and the way they relate to others the better. It has been found that when conflicts arise for example in therapy, how well the conflict can relationally be resolved the better. Conversely, if the client's and therapist's relational patterns clash then the therapeutic endeavor is affected negatively. If, on the other hand, "the extent to which differences and disagreements (can be stated) openly and negotiated so that the therapist (can) flexibly adapt to meet the client's relational patterns" then the alliance is improved, and the outcome is affected more positively.[ix]

In summary, there are approximately ten factors I have identified in the literature that are important from the patient's point of view when they enter the therapeutic arena, *10-Therapist Factors* that need to be present for a good therapeutic experience to take place. This list is not exhaustive however it will be helpful at least as a launch pad for those beginning the therapeutic journey. This initial list of precursory factors needed by the client from the therapist going into the therapy are as follows:

1) For the therapist to display less antagonism and more friendliness, less opposition and more caring, kindlier, warmer tone;
2) For the patient to perceive more support from the therapist, a networking together to feel the backing of the therapist as the patient attempts to take risks to change;
3) For the patient to experience greater comfort from the closeness of the therapist- that the

therapist be able to relate closely with the patient, to tolerate greater interpersonal intimacy

4) For the therapist to have more positive than negative reactions toward the client during the therapy experience;

5) For the therapist to have much more engagement toward the client throughout the therapy;

6) For the therapist to have more effective emotional responsiveness that tends more positively toward the client during the therapeutic experiences shared;

7) For the therapist to possess strong personable attributes such as flexibility, trustworthiness, honesty, respectfulness, confidence, warmth, and to remain interested and open;

8) For the therapist to possess strong skills in exploration, reflection, interpretation, facilitation of affect, and toward attending to a patient's experience;

9) For the therapist to be able to have the ability to attach securely more than anxiously to the patient

10) For the therapist to be relatable to the patient's way of relating, to flexibly be able to adapt to the different ways a patient might relate to the therapist.

These *10-Therapist Factors* will be helpful ways of encouraging you as the reader to approach psychotherapy confidently with a much broader perspective going into the therapeutic setting than you might otherwise if you were to head in "cold turkey," per se, for the first time. Combine these *10-Therapist Factors* with the suggestions you are about to discover from patients in the following case studies who have been there, and you will be closer on your way to a greater start in psychotherapy.

10-THERAPIST FACTORS

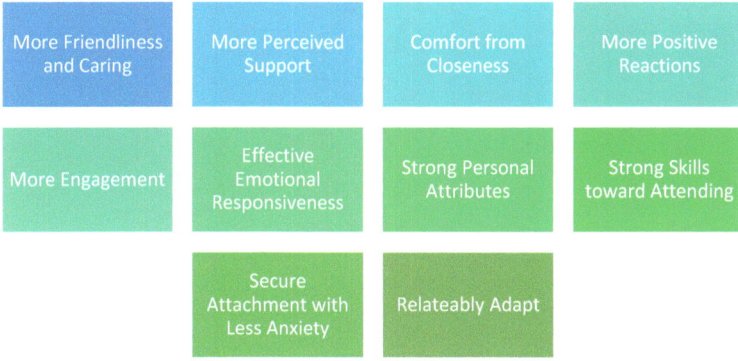

More Friendliness and Caring	More Perceived Support	Comfort from Closeness	More Positive Reactions
More Engagement	Effective Emotional Responsiveness	Strong Personal Attributes	Strong Skills toward Attending
	Secure Attachment with Less Anxiety	Relateably Adapt	

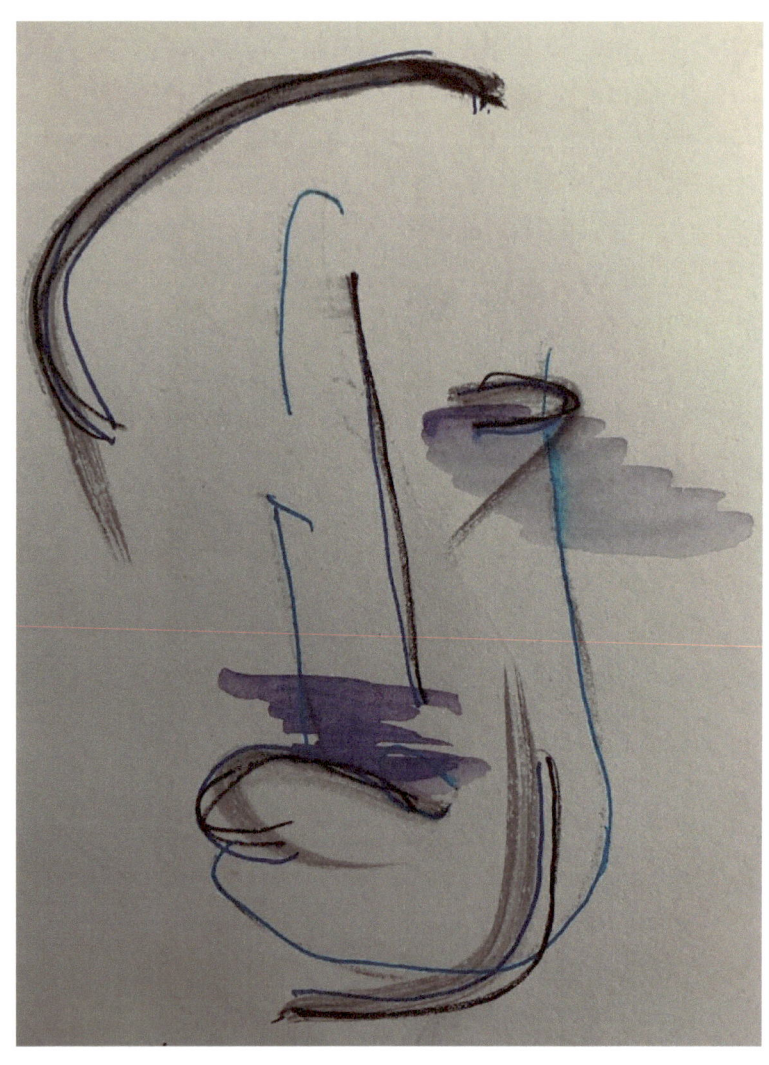

Opening Up

Retitled watercolor on paper canvas with sketch tones
©2006 Dr. Peirsol

CHAPTER 2
CASE STUDIES OF PSYCHOTHERAPY

What I have attempted to do in this chapter is provide specific case studies from live patients sharing their true stories and experiences with psychotherapy. They were each given the same set of questions and the intention again was to illuminate what is important for patients going into the therapeutic arena, sharing what is significant to them in getting the most out of their psychotherapy. The cases vary in terms of gender and age, socioeconomic status, level of education and marital status. Some have never been to therapy before. Others might have been multiple times.

In the following case examples, we explore in greater detail what it is like for patients attending therapy. The questions asked of them were reviewed at the beginning of the book but are also available for your review in each case as you read them. There are several cases in all to draw from and they each have a great deal to pass on to you the reader interested in pursuing psychotherapy for yourself or a loved one.

Read each case study individually and at the end of the chapter is an effort to tie together what the patients have communicated.

CASE STUDY I

This case is a female patient who has never been in therapy before. She is 63 years of age, divorced, currently single, has one grown son and is a professional. She is a pistol and would like to be referred to as either Princess or Diva here in this Case Study.

Question #1. What triggered your awareness that you should seek psychotherapy or the need to see a psychiatrist in the first place? Go into as much detail as you like. What were your initial impressions of needing to see someone, what did you think of psychotherapy then before you even went, and what were you feeling about it before you even got started?

On December 28th 2017, I was diagnosed with cancer.
I was told by my gynecologist that the worst part of his job was telling people they had cancer...I had cancer...I was sent home to wait for the oncologist to call me to set up an appointment for a consultation to map out my treatment. As it was, I had another appointment that same morning with my primary care physician. When I shared with

*him the news I had just received he treated me for
the state of shock I displayed from just learning
that I have cancer! He prescribed an anxiety
medicine to help me stay emotionally level while
working through the next steps in my treatment for
cancer. The medication worked very well but after
a couple of months my primary care physician
recommended seeking the assistance of a therapist
for long term treatment. He explained I would
need the support of a professional in dealing with
cancer and its treatment. I would need to learn
how to manage myself in lieu of relying on
medication solely. I was scared and just reacting
to this uncharted journey I was now traveling. It
made perfect sense to me to have a specialist for
mind, soul, and body...someone professionally and
medically trained to offer support, guidance, and
insight for navigating what was ahead...I was very
encouraged and relieved to know this resource
was made available to me and respected the
integral part it could play in my treatment and
recovery from cancer. Battling cancer was my new
normal and I needed help integrating this reality
into my daily life.*

Question #2. What was it like for you at first, realizing that this is what you need to do, having to find a therapist you liked, your first experience of going to the office, checking in and having that first meeting? Looking back, what was that first session like for you? From your point of view, what was it like being a patient or client in psychotherapy? What was your takeaway and what do you wish you had known then that you know now prior to that first meeting?

I was relieved to know psychotherapy was a resource available to me. My primary care physician made a recommendation for a therapist and scheduled the initial appointment for me. I was not quite certain of what to expect from my first session. I checked in, completed some forms, and waited for my name to be called. As I was sat there, I looked around the waiting area noticing it was simple and understated for a medical office. Then my eye spotted a little framed sign proclaiming, "Look at people, not things." I thought what a nice sentiment, I must be in the right place! My name was called, and I followed the doctor to his office. I took a seat across from his desk anticipating an engaging conversation about my situation and how his expertise recommendations would help me manage my cancer diagnosis. He immediately began to ask me the regular preliminary questions for a new patient as he typed and stared into the computer screen. As he completed his inquiries, I was remembering the framed sign in the waiting room and I was excited anticipating the doctor was going turn his attention to me exclusively. To my dismay, he continued to stare into the computer and asked me what made me most upset about having cancer? My voice broke with emotion as I responded, "Talking about it." But still no eye contact just type, type, type. At the end of it all he prescribed medication and informed me that I would be assigned to see one of the practicing therapists. I thanked him and left chuckling to myself as I recalled my experience against the sign from the waiting room. I left the initial meeting less than satisfied with the results. I really hoped my next appointment would produce a different impression. Not knowing what to expect during that first visit perhaps contributed to my disappointment.

Question #3. What made you decide to go back after the first session? What came of the initial stages of your treatment/therapy and what do you recall most about your experience early on? Looking back is there anything you wish you would have known or done differently now looking back on that initial period?

I returned for my 2nd appointment on the promise I was seeing someone different. My initial visit with Dr. P was relaxed, calm, and attentive! I sat on a very comfortable oversized sofa across from his desk and he faced me as we engaged in conversation! I was still a little nervous about what the sessions were going to entail but I was comfortable in the setting. Dr P was easy to talk with and put me at ease with his warm smile, kind eyes and pleasant demeanor. It was evident he wanted me to feel comfortable. We chatted and I gained a better understanding of what to expect from our sessions. Upon leaving I felt more confident and encouraged, more hopeful. Here was someone who wanted to be part of my journey, to help guide and equip me with skills and insights to manage living my life with cancer.

Questions #4. What did you discover along the way, things about yourself that you might not have expected, things you liked and things you didn't? What do you remember most about the most difficult part(s) of the therapy experience? Looking back, what were some of the initial changes you started to make as a result of the therapy? How did your point of view of psychotherapy start to change during this process and what do you think of it now looking back?

During the course of therapy, I discovered I was not quite as strong as I believed in some aspects of managing myself but stronger than I realized in others. Maintaining an emotional steadiness was very difficult which surprised me because I prided myself on being in control of my emotional self. My level of insecurities increased in the face of this realization...where was my strength to maintain emotional steadiness...was I too weak to push forward? But on the other hand, I had a fierce resolve to stay positive while undergoing treatment for cancer.

I did not like the roller coaster of emotions but was quite surprised with my determination to keep up the fight, to remain hopeful and positive. This resolve also became increasingly exhausting. As a woman of faith, I was alarmed at the feeling of being distant from God after my diagnosis. I understand God did not move but rather the deep trauma of learning I had cancer shook my certainty that God was still close by. My therapist shared techniques to help neutralize my anxiety. From meditation to embracing my feelings as a familiar friend, albeit a challenging friend. The more I focused on learned practices instead of the problems connected with my cancer diagnosis, the calmer and steadier I remained and for longer periods of time.

I believe therapy to be a medical approach for addressing issues of the mind and soul. I knew that proper mental focus and practiced repetitions would train my mind to default to a more rational place in order to continue positive progress. I have realized this takes time and is a process that involves an imperfect vessel. But I am still standing strong.

Question #5. What made the therapy work for you? What did you learn most about yourself that was a surprise and what changed for you, in life, your relationships, etc. in the process of being a patient or client in psychotherapy? Looking back was there anything about yourself you discovered that you wished you had known before going to therapy and what difference do you think that may have made in your life if you had known it prior to therapy?

I believe therapy works for me because I trust my therapist. Trust allows me to be transparent and honest concerning what is in my heart and on my mind. One area I wish I had a better understanding of and dealt with more effectively was the trauma I suffered during my marriage. I thought I had the experiences all tied up and placed on a shelf never to be opened again.... until an incident triggered the ugly memories and they surfaced during a session. It was upsetting to realize that I had not worked through this trauma and now felt a fear inside that I described as a "jello feeling".

Looking back, I should have entered therapy after my divorce. Therapy would have afforded me stronger confidence and esteem in regard to my self-worth. Although I believe I possess a very gregarious personality, thoughts of myself as damaged goods now that I had cancer seemed to invade my mind daily. How could anyone love me now?

I believe I could have lessened the feelings of worthlessness after my cancer diagnosis if had entered therapy after experiencing the trauma in my marriage.

But I am working now to mend my heart and heal my mind so I can fight strong against this disease with every fiber of my being. Mind, body, and soul function optimally as a whole...independently they are fragmented...

QUESTION #6. Looking back on your therapy experience, thinking about others that could have learned from what you experienced as a result of therapy, what is there you would want to tell them if you could that maybe as a result of what you learned they would be able to avoid the difficulties you experienced? What is it that you would want to tell them about psychotherapy that you wished you knew before now so that maybe they too could get the most out of it if they chose to go?

One of the lessons and messages I would like others to know about therapy is start early and go often to sessions!

We are wired so delicately and magnificently that we should not solely rely on our own capabilities to filter life's experiences through the prism of our fractured reasoning and rational. Finding a therapist who shares your values and ideals coupled with their professional medical training is the best combination for seeking feedback and direction along your life's journey.

Question #7. What are the most important things you have learned as a result of your experience in psychotherapy? What do want to be sure others know from your point of view about your experience in psychotherapy, what you want to give back if you had the chance to tell them now?

The important thing I learned as a result of my experience in psychotherapy is being in therapy is ok! Often people are afraid of a stigma being attached to being in therapy sessions.
Also, you are not replacing your thoughts, opinions, and reasoning with that of your therapist. But rather view your therapists as a facilitator of insight and guidance, a partner in developing healthy practices, thought processes, and habits designed to optimize your life's journey. Not just a journey of survival but rather a journey of flourishing and blooming into a life well lived; a life measured in inspiration for yourself and others!

Always strive to be your best so you can invest your best into others!

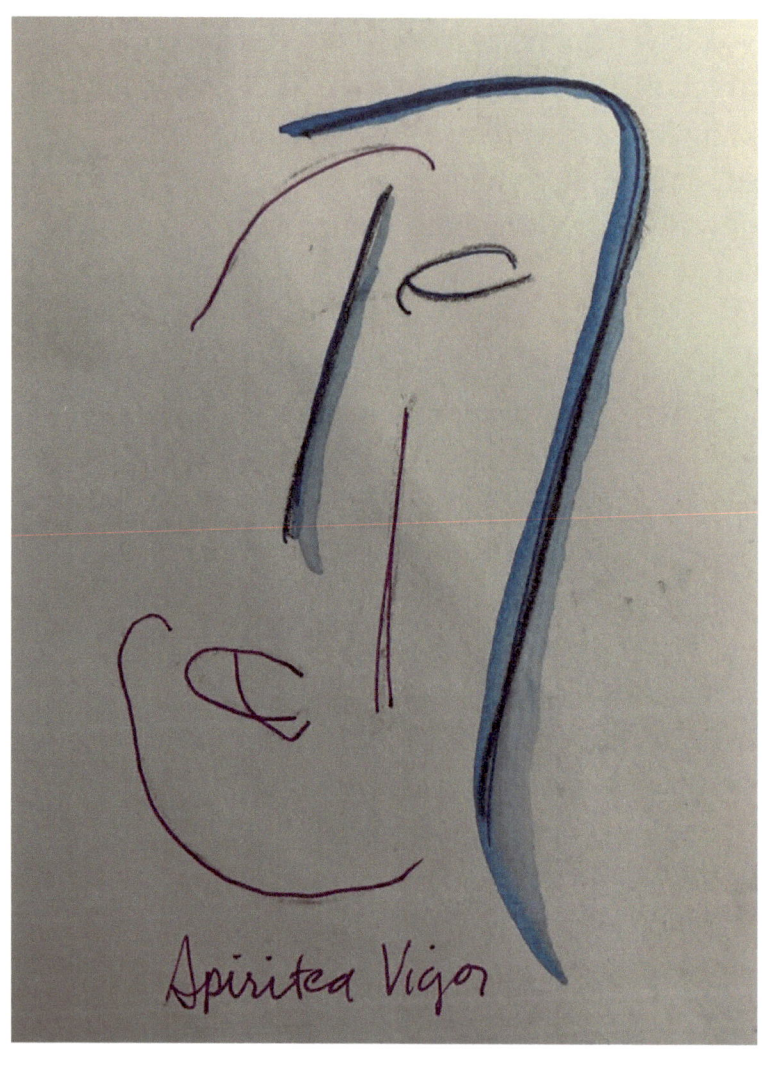

Watercolor on paper canvas with sketch tones
©2006 Dr. Peirsol

CASE STUDY II

This case is of a father is married and has one daughter and one son, the son is the one he brought into treatment.

Question #1. What triggered your awareness that you should seek psychotherapy or the need to see a psychiatrist in the first place? Go into as much detail as you like. What were your initial impressions of needing to see someone, what did you think of psychotherapy then before you even went, and what were you feeling about it before you even got started?

I never felt like I ever needed it, but when the addiction situation came up with my teenage son I was searching for answers and realized I couldn't find the answers I needed on my own.

Question #2. What was it like for you at first, realizing that this is what you need to do, having to find a therapist you liked, your first experience of going to the office, checking in and having that first meeting? Looking back, what was that first session like for you? From your point of view, what was it like being a patient or client in psychotherapy? What was your takeaway and what do you wish you had known then that you know now prior to that first meeting?

The first meeting was a relief. My wife and I liked the therapist and our son seemed to like him too. He answered many of the questions we were having. Mostly we were concerned about mental illness from drug abuse, but he assured us it was a drug induced psychosis with schizophrenic symptoms as opposed to mental illness. That was a big relief.

Question #3. What made you decide to go back after the first session? What came of the initial stages of your treatment/therapy and what do you recall most about your experience early on? Looking back is there anything you wish you would have known or done differently now looking back on that initial period?

We felt like we were making progress and our son seemed to be responding to the therapy. My wife also decided to get some individual counseling after the ordeal of having our son baker-acted the week before Christmas. We also were counseled together to help us cope as a family. We kept our daughter out of it, although I wish I got her some counseling to help her cope with her brother's errant ways and really mistreating her by not paying any attention to her during those years of his addiction.

Question #4. What did you discover along the way, things about yourself that you might not have expected, things you liked and things you didn't? What do you remember most about the most difficult part(s) of the therapy experience? Looking back, what were some of the initial changes you started to make as a result of the therapy? How did your point of view of psychotherapy start to change during this process and what do you think of it now looking back?

I don't think our marriage would have lasted without the therapy. It helped us take the blame off ourselves and focus more on the disruptive behaviors our son's addiction that was inflicting all kinds of discord for the family. It helped us to understand the underlying reasons for the addiction and to put more energy into healing aspects of the therapy rather than show anger towards the behavior. It helped us see the addiction as a sickness, rather than some reckless, selfish behavior, although it certainly seemed like it at first and so that is why we were angry at him and ourselves for letting this horrible thing happen to our beautiful son.

Question #5. What made the therapy work for you? What did you learn most about yourself that was a surprise and what changed for you, in life, your relationships, etc. in the process of being a patient or client in psychotherapy? Looking back was there anything about yourself you discovered that you wished you had known before going to therapy and what difference do you think that may have made in your life if you had known it prior to therapy?

I think I learned how to become a stronger father figure for my son. Towards the conclusion of his addiction (15 years later) I was monitoring his behavior on a daily basis. I never would have done that prior to getting family counseling. I think it really did make a difference in his recovery and ultimately, he looks up to more as a role model for him now that he is a parent. It's been win/win for both of us.

Question #6. Looking back on your therapy experience, thinking about others that could have learned from what you experienced as a result of therapy, what is there you would want to tell them if you could that maybe as a result of what you learned they would be able to avoid the difficulties you experienced? What is it that you would want to tell them about psychotherapy that you wished you knew before now so that maybe they too could get the most out of it if they chose to go?

Not to lean too much on the therapist to resolve the issues at hand. Take an active role in overcoming things that get in the way, show courage and be strong about it. Whining will not get you the results you and your therapist want. The determination to change things must come from within. Always have hope, have heart and never give up. In other words, be prepared to slay the dragon.

Question #7. What are the most important things you have learned as a result of your experience in psychotherapy? What do want to be sure others know from your point of view about your experience in psychotherapy, what you want to give back if you had the chance to tell them now?

No one said it would be easy. Real change doesn't happen overnight. Look for the little signs of improvement and be encouraged by that along the way. Have patience, show love and above all expect to have setbacks. Relapses are part of the process of change. I wish I had known that early on. I don't think I would have felt so discouraged each time it happened. There is no such thing as failure when it comes to healing an addicted person. All you can really do is have faith, show compassion, and hope they come through it all, one day at a time for the rest of their lives.

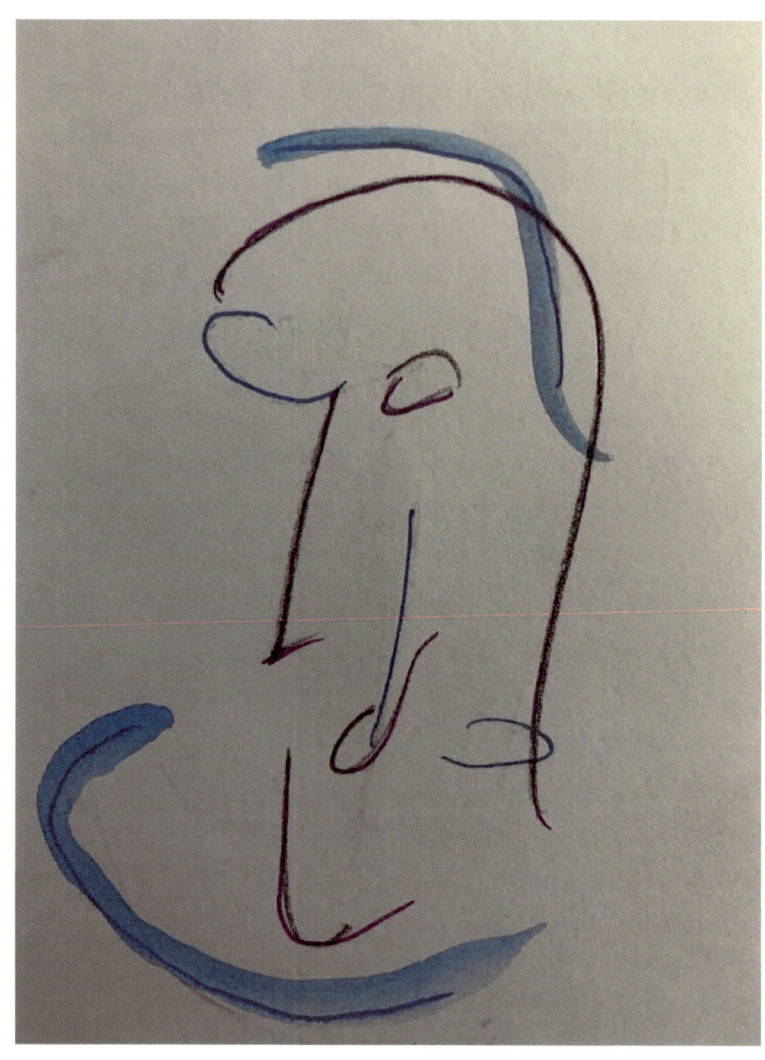

Untitled watercolor on paper canvas with sketch tones
©2006 Dr. Peirsol

CASE STUDY III

This case is a 48-year old male who is in his 3rd marriage, has three (3) children and one stepdaughter. He is a professional IT Specialist with a current diagnosis Bipolar I. He is an avid hunter and angler, is a southerner and is currently continuing his studies as a Programmer.

Question #1. What triggered your awareness that you should seek psychotherapy or the need to see a psychiatrist in the first place? Go into as much detail as you like. What were your initial impressions of needing to see someone, what did you think of psychotherapy then before you even went, and what were you feeling about it before you even got started?

I was hanging on by a thread and that thread was about to break. I was in my first year of having my own business and was making a real mess of things. I had just lost my father and I was all over the map, the pain was real and most days I just didn't want to exist at all. I couldn't think or sit still long enough to get anything done even though I felt like I was, at least while I was doing it. It was only at the end of the day when I truly realized I hadn't accomplished anything at all. My wife

finally came to me and told me that she felt like I really needed to see someone, and advised me to see a therapist so I googled therapists in my area and found one that I thought I liked and that the insurance would help pay for. But I didn't go right away, for the next two months, I kept putting it off, I thought it was all a racket of some sort to take my money. "How could talking to a complete stranger help me in any way"? I pondered this question for quite some time until I knew that something was certainly wrong, something I could not handle on my own. But, was it really possible a complete stranger could help me? I wasn't optimistic in the least.

Question #2. What was it like for you at first, realizing that this is what you need to do, having to find a therapist you liked, your first experience of going to the office, checking in and having that first meeting? Looking back, what was that first session like for you? From your point of view, what was it like being a patient or client in psychotherapy? What was your take away and what do you wish you had known then that you know now prior to that first meeting?

I lived with anger, anxiety and times of the uncertainty of my being for forty-three years, I thought it was just a part of life. Why did everything seem so much worse now? I didn't understand. My father had just passed unexpectedly and I was taking it very hard but I could barely write an email, the anger was out of control and there were a lot of days where I couldn't get out of bed. I lied to my wife and those around me and told them I was sick— I thought maybe I was but I knew it had to be more than that. I knew that my life was falling apart and that if something didn't get fixed soon, I was going to lose everything. I didn't want to talk to a stranger about my problems, it was embarrassing. I was brought up that a man handles his own affairs, to man up, cowboy the fuck up, and just get on with it, but my wife told me that kind of mentality was total bullshit and that I needed help from someone who knew how to help me. I realized at that moment I had never really helped myself at all no matter how many times I believed I was manning up, and that I had to get help. I walked into the therapist's office for the first time, closed up as tight as a locked door. I wanted to be open with her, truly open but I didn't know how. I Chose a woman therapist because for some reason I felt she would be more easy to talk to. My first session was nerve racking but my therapist was great. She made me feel comfortable and that was a huge plus glad I listened because that is where it all began to change for me. My fifth therapist is where I found out that I have bipolar disorder. Another thing that I found out and paid dearly emotionally was when choosing a therapist to make sure that they fit you, if not ditch them and find someone who does, you will be thankful you did in the long run.

Question #3. What made you decide to go back after the first session? What came of the initial stages of your treatment/therapy and what do you recall most about your experience early on? Looking back is there anything you wish you would have known or done differently now looking back on that initial period?

After seeing four different therapists over the course of two years, it was really hard to get interested in looking for another one. When I did go it was to see a psychiatrist, not just another therapist, it was he, the psychiatrist that set me up with the therapist that I am seeing presently. I almost got up and left on the first visit but made myself stay, and I'm thankful that I did because it has been the best psychotherapy to date for me. After the first session, I was ready and eager to go back, curious as much as eager I would say. Curious I think because I couldn't believe that anyone cared enough to really listen. Most of the other therapists seemed to already know what I was going to say before I said it as they had already lived my life somehow. It immediately made me think that the whole psychotherapy thing was a sham, a scam to get your money. After a few sessions, the doctor diagnosed me with Bipolar disorder. I was forty-six at the time. It was difficult to deal with the diagnosis initially and I became obsessed with the disorder instead of getting better. Looking back, I wish I would have put more emphasis on moving forward and getting better and not allow the disorder label to consume me.

Question #4. What did you discover along the way, things about yourself that you might not have expected, things you liked and things you didn't? What do you remember most about the most difficult part(s) of the therapy experience? Looking back, what were some of the initial changes you started to make as a result of the therapy? How did your point of view of psychotherapy start to change during this process and what do you think of it now looking back?

Having the correct diagnosis is paramount to really knowing what to do next. Finding a therapist that gets you, but lets you talk and sees you for who you are is a must for healing, dealing with everyday life, and just plain existing. For forty-six years I lived without the proper diagnosis and it cost me dearly, not just financially but emotionally as well. As my therapist began to see the real me, not just the person that was hidden underneath the shame, regret, and fear of complete and utter failure, I also began to see me and I began to wonder— "could it be that I am really not all the things that the voice in my head tells me I am"? For the first time in my life I was beginning to believe that there was hope, that there was a better tomorrow and that I might just be okay, maybe even better than okay. I found out that I am a good person with a huge heart and I liked that, I also found out that I am jealous and not very good at making decisions, prone to vicious cycles of anger for no reason at all, and no matter how good I felt there was always that nagging feeling or unrelenting voice keeping me up to date on how much of a failure I was. The most difficult part of the therapy for me was having to let everything inside out for my therapist to see, mainly because most of the things I had tucked away so far inside that I had purposely forgotten them. Even in my darkest times when I want to die and leave all the

*pain behind, I hear my therapist's voice telling me
that I am not a failure no matter what my brain is
telling me. The turning point that changed the way
I see psychotherapy really happened when I heard
that voice above the voice in my brain telling me to
kill myself because it would be a service to
everyone around me. I knew then the impact of
having someone trained in psychotherapy to talk to
was often for me the defining difference in staying
alive or becoming a statistic.*

Question #5. What made the therapy work for
you? What did you learn most about yourself that
was a surprise and what changed for you, in life,
your relationships, etc. in the process of being a
patient or client in psychotherapy? Looking back
was there anything about yourself you discovered
that you wished you had known before going to
therapy and what difference do you think that may
have made in your life if you had known it prior to
therapy?

*I think what made the therapy work for me was
that I finally reached the point to where I had to
trust someone and it made me feel like someone
really cared what happened to me. Learning to
trust myself and others was huge for me, it opened
many doors that I had closed before and it led me*

to start believing in myself again. No matter how bad the episodes of bipolar, I felt more grounded than before and a little more in control of my life. I wished I would have known about the disorder many years before and had learned how to trust myself and others instead of shutting myself and everyone out, I am sure it would have made a difference in everything, from career choices to relationships.

Question #6. Looking back on your therapy experience, thinking about others that could have learned from what you experienced as a result of therapy, what is there you would want to tell them if you could that maybe as a result of what you learned they would be able to avoid the difficulties you experienced? What is it that you would want to tell them about psychotherapy that you wished you knew before now so that maybe they too could get the most out of it if they chose to go?

If I could help anyone from suffering the pain that I have suffered, I would say to them that it's not easy and it's okay to be scared, it's also completely okay not to be strong, you cannot do this alone. Mental illness is real, and it will leave you feeling powerless and if left untreated, it can and will destroy your life. You must talk to someone about what you are experiencing, trust someone who is trained to help you, and as much as it is humanly possible, be completely open to your therapist, it not only speeds up the process incorrect diagnosis but in helping you get back to living a better life. Medication if needed and prescribed by a doctor helps the part of the brain that is causing the illness but cognitive therapy by a trained and licensed therapist helps you understand it all a little better so that you learn to know yourself. No matter how much you might believe the lie, you are not alone, someone wants to help you, take that first step for yourself and the ones you love, and change your life for the better. Without professional help lives are ruined, dreams are put on hold and some really beautiful souls succumb to the lies of depression and wind up a statistic. Suicide only leaves more pain, guilt and suffering behind for the ones that love you. If I would have known years ago what I know today about psychotherapy, I wouldn't have waited one single minute to make an appointment and go talk to a therapist. I lost years, careers, relationships, and dreams to the mental disorder called bipolar, but through therapy both cognitive and medication, I am slowly but surely taking back my life from its deathly grasp.

Question #7. What are the most important things you have learned as a result of your experience in psychotherapy? What do want to be sure others know from your point of view about your experience in psychotherapy, what you want to give back if you had the chance to tell them now?

I am not a failure nor a mistake. You are not a failure nor a mistake, and there is nothing wrong with who you are, it is a loop in your brain that is telling you the lie. It is not the truth no matter how bad it hurts or makes you feel. It is all real, the pain, the guilt and the moments but it doesn't have to define you. Therapists are trained to see you for who you really are, they are on the outside looking in so they have a clear view of who you are. Being open with my therapist and trusting the process is the only way to tame the beast and allow yourself to really live your life not the disorder's script for your life. I admit it has been extremely difficult at times to trust the process and I have fallen off the wagon many times but I went back and that's what matters. Every day is a new challenge but through treatment and therapy, I have started my own business, have a great relationship with my wife and kids since my diagnosis. This wouldn't have been even a long shot at being possible without professional help. You can do this, you can take back your life starting today! Don't give this shit another second of your life, call someone today, make an appointment and show up, you will be glad you did.

CASE STUDY IV

I am a nurse and have worked with psychiatric patients in some capacity all of my nursing career. So, the idea of going to a therapist never bothered me because I knew the right one could definitely make a difference in your life. Going the first day was a little scary and I'll tell you why. One day my husband of 46 years packed up his belongings (taking 9 hrs. to do it) and left. I was devastated! We had been happy, both retired, have always enjoyed each other, have common interests, so it was something I could not grasp no matter how hard I tried. After he returned with no explanation, no "I'm sorry" - nothing. I decided we had to see someone because I wanted and needed answers. We found Dr. Peirsol and made an appt. Yes, I was nervous because I didn't know if he would be understanding and help us to find the reason my husband left and what part I had played in this. I deserved an explanation and apology. But most of all we needed to find out what was going on in my husband's mind that had made him leave to begin with. I actually looked forward to seeing a *psychologist because my husband had been depressed and had mood swings. As I said earlier if you get the right therapist then seeing one is very helpful. It's important to **get a therapist who listens to you**, doesn't talk all the time, hears what you are saying and reserves judgement, especially with a couple. As we checked in at the office, I was a little uneasy because I was embarrassed even though I know better than to think someone would be labeling us as "crazy." As we entered the therapist's office it was dimly lit, a little chilly, my husband and I sat on a couch. It was very calming. The therapist made us feel very comfortable, he gave each of us a time to explain what had happened and express our feelings. He quickly learned how to re-direct my husband who sometimes gets carried away in his stories. Each session my husband was sent home with an assignment related to his feelings that he needed to work on. I was there to help him. As we left that first session I felt as if the therapist really understood and was going to help both of us. Of course, we wanted to return because as it turned out we had a lot of work to do on our relationship. There were times when my husband would go alone and then I would have a session without him. Those were very helpful because sometimes you have a question or a subject that you don't wish to discuss in front of your spouse. I did learn something about me and we both learned things about my husband and his early childhood. Things* *he had never discussed and did not want to, but the realization of how much this had influenced our relationship was very important in our healing. At home we were able to discuss these things without being disagreeable.*

There were many times during therapy that I cried, my husband cried, we cried together. But I never felt uncomfortable while shedding the tears. In looking back, I wish I had known more of my husband's early childhood, I knew some but not all. He has always been a private person and his answer is always, "I'm ok." I discovered that in spite of my happy nature I could be very demanding at times. No, I knew it all along, but I learned that I had to curb my demands and the tone of my voice. It worked. We also learned that if we had an issue with the other person we stopped right then and dealt with it. This was great.

*I think what made the therapy work for us is that we did our "homework" and also **put into action** the relationship tools which we had learned. It took me a long time to trust that he would not leave again. It was over a year before my heart could really love him again. We have always taken our wedding vows very seriously, so we had to get over this hump.*

My husband finally said he was sorry and apologized for hurting me. I must tell you that my husband had been diagnosed with Vascular Brain Disease prior to leaving me and us going to therapy. He has the same symptoms as Alzheimer's dis. but his is due to brain shrinkage. I had to finally understand that he felt overwhelmed, thought I was nagging, and didn't see a way out but to leave.

One of the important things I learned is to stop and discuss an issue before it becomes a full-blown argument. I have also learned, and this was not easy at all for me, to be more patient with my husband. He is a good man, a wonderful spouse and father. I cannot image my life without him. But I can be impatient.

I would strongly encourage anyone having marital disagreements (and who doesn't) to seek some help. There is nothing embarrassing about going. I think most men think they are too "macho" to go to therapy, but it is a very helpful and can give any couple some wonderful tools with which to work. When we got married now, 48 years ago, there was no such thing as pre-marital counseling, but I would strongly encourage any young couple to go prior to getting married.

I think the key to any successful counseling experience is having the correct therapist - ours was wonderful, I could tell by his looks that he understood my pain even though I didn't say much about it. He was always calm and gave us time to answer questions, made sure each session that he asked us how our progress was going and then asked how we were doing. That gave us a chance to begin a conversation. We have now been married for 48 years and looking forward to fifty (and many more). I would like to tell people that each of us **at some time on our lives needs some outside help**. *Most people don't get the help they need for many reasons, but it is* **very cleansing** *to have a good therapist and get some things out of your brain and heart.*

Just a side note, don't know if you can use it or not.

I was a nurse manager for a company. I was 6 months from being 100% vested and I was not going to give it up plus I would also get 4 weeks' vacation/year. There were only two of us in the office and I was the one in charge. The other lady was very argumentative, not easy to get along with, thought she was always right, and on and on. She made the work environment very thick because of our inability to get along. Our boss in another city told us to have a morning meeting every day and see if that would help. Of course, it didn't work because she never had time to stop and meet. I was at my wits end, so I called the Mental Health branch of our health insurance. They referred me to a lady psychologist. I went to see her, explaining the issues at work and asking how I could better handle it. She informed me that I needed to quit. Well, it's not hard to believe that I left, very discouraged and in tears. She was a real disappointment. It turned me against therapy for a long time. I did not quit my job and with some restructuring that occurred in our office she finally quit. I am sure you know that I did not shed any tears over that. Sometimes it's better to listen to your own heart and mind than do something someone tells you to.

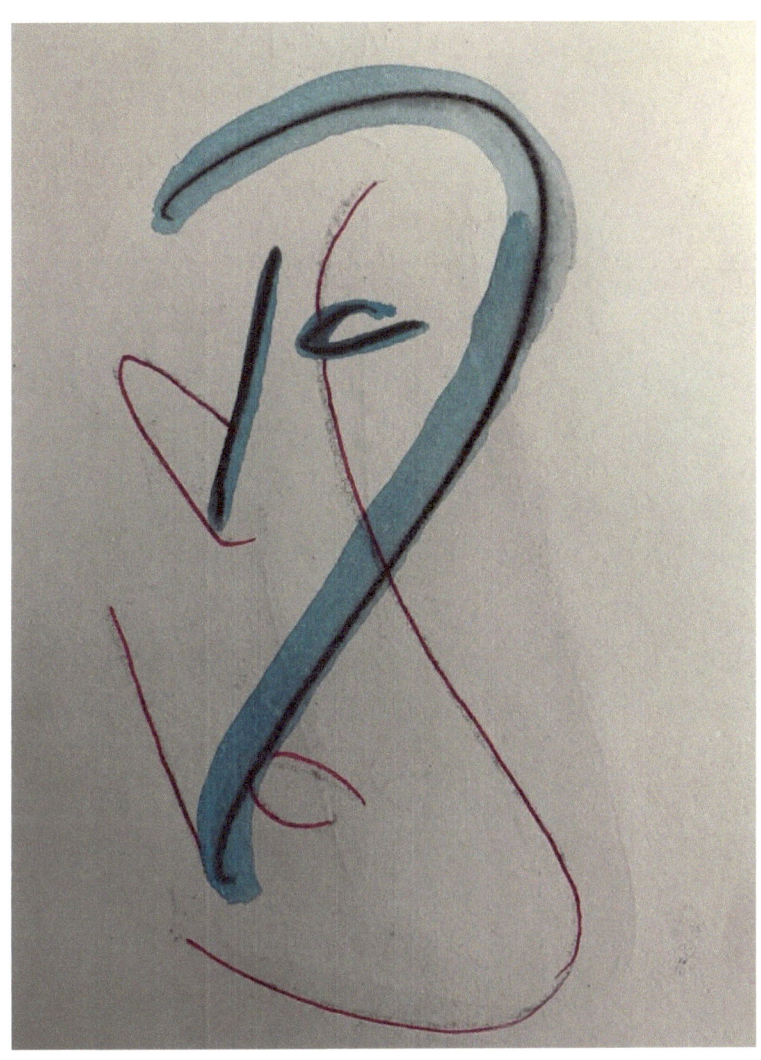

Awareness. Keen Insight

Retitled watercolor on paper canvas with sketch tones
©2019 Dr. Peirsol

CHAPTER 3
FINDING YOUR WAY IN THERAPY

In this chapter, I intend to explore the dynamics from each of the case studies presented, to make an effort to take each set of questions and provide a brief summary of each of the sets of questions so an overview of the case examples can shed light on what patients' point of views may be about psychotherapy. What are the takeaways for us as the readers to be able to consider for ourselves as we, too, look at the benefits of psychotherapy from a patient's point of view?

In reading each case study, it is apparent each experience with psychotherapy has its differences; however, each one is relieved they started the therapy. As much of a hesitation at first appears to have been exceeded by the relief they felt once they started. They each had their own considerations at the start of seeking help however it seems in the end that it is better not to hesitate too long; that the sooner you get started the better.

In looking at the first set of questions, *No. 1*, asked in the case studies, it primarily focused upon first impression of the idea of going to therapy. There is a range of reaction to the notion of going to psychotherapy initially, it is not similar for any of the cases, each is different. The responses range from "psychotherapy" being a welcomed addition to their situation, to feeling forced into it somewhat reluctantly but willingly especially for the welfare of a loved one, to totally disregarding it as a racket and a sham.

This range of reaction to the notion of psychotherapy depicts a great deal of those who show up in my office for the first time, feeling relieved to be there on the one hand or reluctant at best to being there foremost. I do not recall anyone necessarily showing up in my office "thrilled to be there that first day of therapy." I think the lack luster of the thrill however in many cases is the fact they have a burden to share that bothers them most rather than the fact they are seeking psychotherapy initially. The feeling of "Why me?" is more at play than the question of "Why psychotherapy?" for the most part. Generally speaking, those who show up in the office are those that want help, so they are looking for answers to their problems. Children and adolescents brought in by their parents have tended to be the most resistant to this initial stage of the process of therapy.

With this, "What would you say your impressions are of psychotherapy today as the reader of this book, especially those of you that might not have tried it yet before?" Considering your circumstances, what have the reflections of these cases had on your own impressions of psychotherapy at the outset?

The next set of questions, *No. 2* from the list of case study questions, earmarks that first session and what you can expect it to be like. From the cases, just like in question one, the first session experiences varied as well, from disappointment to great relief depending upon the connection made with the therapist. Thus, the ability to relate at first with the therapist is a crucial element coming in. Ultimately, the better the therapist can relate to you the better that first session will go.

There really is no way to prejudge what that first session with a therapist will be like; however, you can double check with others about the way the therapist relates to their patients by asking around even if you ask the front desk staff at the therapist's office. Or, better yet, ask the therapist yourself if you actually get to talk to them beforehand. Come right out directly and ask how they relate to their patients. Are they sociable in their sessions, do they relate well to others, and will they be able to make you feel comfortable getting started?

The next set of questions, *No. 3,* are very important because the momentum at the start is very important when getting going in the therapy process. If it starts out well, it likely ends well. Thankfully in each of the cases presented, they all seem to get off to a good start. They ranged from instilling hope in that first session, to creating results in another, and helping one to become more curious about the process in the next. *Hope filled with curiosity and results is not a bad start for therapy.*

Thus, when you go into your first session it might be a good rule of thumb to seek more *hope* about your situation. "Will this situation I am in turn around? Can it turn around?" and "Will it get better?" are some of the questions that might be considered when seeking hope from that initial session. Hope can come in the form of not being alone facing one's issues, and hope can be instilled just by knowing that someone is there for you in dealing with what concerns you.

Curiosity, on the other hand, can take some effort; however, just the mere fact one might seek help is in itself a curious endeavor. So, to become more curious about the process might require more inquiry on your end coming in. "Wondering what the process is like?" and "How it all works to get better?" are some of the questions one might ask to instill more curiosity as a result of an initial session. With renewed curiosity comes more motivation; and, feeling more motivated is really important when it comes to getting started in psychotherapy. With motivation, one is willing to take risks for example; and, being in therapy itself is a huge risk. The idea here is all about the notion of change and with any new changes comes challenges which always require risk taking because with change is always having to face the unknown.

Results on the other hand, keep in mind, at least from the initial few sessions, can come in the form of simply becoming more informed as to whether or not you are okay- it can be in seeing one become more responsive to the situation, or even less responsive; or, it can come by feeling a change as a result of new insight. Results vary for each person and could be as simple as feeling heard, feeling cared for, and or even just being listened to. All in all, though, it is important to consider results from a more tangible vantage point, looking instead for outcomes that you can walk away with, seeing results that come with a renewed curiosity and hope is a worthwhile guideline to knowing whether or not the psychotherapy is working at first. Thus, it is okay to ask you therapist to help you walk away with tangible results at the start. This can come in the form of those listed here or in multiple different ways. Just make sure whatever way you decide will work for is tangible enough when you walk away from your initial meetings in psychotherapy.

The fourth set of questions, *No. 4,* gets at the unexpected that can come from psychotherapy.

From realizing on the one hand "I am not as strong as I thought I was" to "I am stronger than I imagined" or that "the therapy not only saved my marriage, but it saved my life" sort of scenario is in effect life altering altogether. Thus, at least from these cases, one can expect psychotherapy to be just that: life altering in its application. Expect the unexpected with positive outliers. In other words, anticipate something more to happen than you might initially expect. Something good is going to happen and it is going to be better at a minimum in your life as a result of going to psychotherapy. With this, it is important to consider "Why wait to start?" If in each case, there was a positively impactful result that was a welcomed surprise then it could be considered this could possibly happen for you. It can be assumed; psychotherapy brings with it the assurance of something better as a result. It might not be everything you think but it will be better as a result. This is reassuring to hear especially for those that might be reluctant to try. From the patient's perspective, they are saying psychotherapy is beneficial in ways that might not have every been anticipated.

The questions in the *No. 5* set are inquiring about what might have been discovered as a result of psychotherapy and whether or not this discovery could have made a difference sooner had one gone to psychotherapy earlier on in their life.

Unanimously, each case study suggests something was discovered they could have benefitted from had they known about it sooner in their lives. The impact of a previous divorce, the newly established role modeling as a father, the issues of spouse, the sense of belief in oneself, all could have benefited each individual differently had such been explored in their lives sooner. The takeaway is we all have things to uncover we might not notice just yet that could be helped along if we took the time to address them in psychotherapy. The key is to practice what one learns in session however when learning occurs. Do your homework one spouse said emphatically. Put into action what you learn early on. We may not know exactly what that is just yet but there is something we each have to offer up that could improve if we took the time to consider psychotherapy.

The questions in set *No. 6* consider what one can take from one's therapy experience to offer to someone else for having done it. The cases together specifically suggest *12-Takeaways to offer from Psychotherapy*. They are listed below and presented in *Figure 1*.

1) "go early"
2) and "go often"
3) "seek feedback and direction along your life's journey"
4) it's a "win/win"
5) "it's also completely okay not to be strong, you cannot do this alone"
6) "Mental illness is real, and it will leave you feeling powerless and if left untreated it can and will destroy your life"
7) "You must talk to someone about what you are experiencing…it help(s) you get back to living a better life"
8) "Medication …helps"
9) "take that first step for yourself and the ones you love, and change your life for the better"
10) Do not "wait one single minute to make an appointment and go talk to a therapist"
11) "through therapy…(you can) "slowly but surely (take) back (your) life."
12) do your homework: put into action what you have learned

TWELVE-TAKEAWAYS FROM PSYCHOTHERAPY

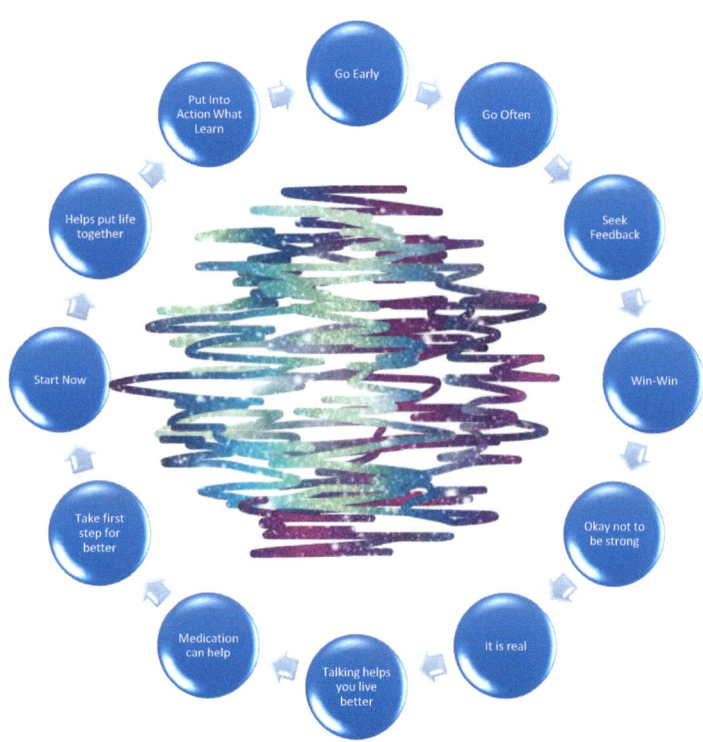

Figure 1

In review of the *12-Takeaways*, there are four primary principles or rules of thumb that can be drawn initially from this list. Some of them can be taken at face value and others postulated. They are presented in *Figure 2* below for your review and consideration.

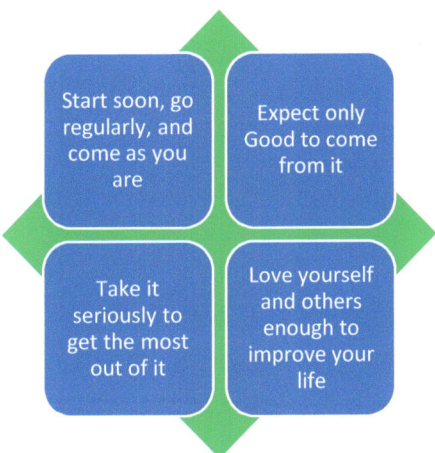

Figure 2: **Rules of Thumb** for psychotherapy

The last set of questions, **No. 7**, address what patients want to be sure to tell the audience about their experience overall with psychotherapy. In this type of conclusion, the cases have indicated multiple messages to us as the reader. One is to avoid the stigma of going by accepting the fact that it is "Okay" to be in psychotherapy; that it is not a bad thing to do for yourself or that we all need advice at one time or another in life. To realize as part of psychotherapy you still get to be yourself and are not expected to give up the way you think or feel but rather improve upon what you think or feel. Therapy is a place where you can receive needed guidance to improve the quality of your life as you know it, the idea that therapy can be a means to "flourishing and blooming into a life well lived; a life measured in inspiration for yourself and others!"

Another message is to accept that change takes time in psychotherapy, that it "doesn't happen overnight!" and to look for the small changes along the way as a sign of encouragement as one way to look at the psychotherapeutic process, with the understanding that there will be "setbacks" along the way. "Relapses are part of the process of change…(and) there is no such thing as failure when it comes to healing."

Another case study encourages others with the message that the struggle one faces "doesn't have to define you"; that the difficulties and the setbacks are all a part of the process of mental health concerns. They go so far to say that "being open with (the) therapist and trusting the process is the only way to tame the beast and allow yourself to really live your life." In addition, they reiterate the importance of not waiting, to go ahead and get started in the process, that one should "make an appointment and show up, you will be glad you did" notion.

In effect, psychotherapy has much greater benefits than the drawbacks one may typically associate with it. For as much as one might feel it is just for people with problems, there are countless individuals who have found a new lease on life as a result of its benefits. For as much time as it might take to complete the process, there is so much time wasted headed in the wrong direction before ever learning there is an alternative route to consider. For as many doubts as there might be about the process of psychotherapy, there are countless stories that prove the process to be worthwhile and helpful over and above all the frustrations that may appear to come with it.

In this next chapter, I want to elaborate upon some guidelines to consider when one begins the therapeutic process, all in an effort to ensure that the individual seeking counsel can get the most out of it from the start. These particular Guidelines are gathered from the literature and elaborated upon as a result of years of experience watching and participating with patients in psychotherapy. At first glance, some of the Guidelines can be taken at face value; but, it will be important to understanding why the Guideline is there to help facilitate a more therapeutic experience for all involved.

These recommendations are pretty forthright and forthcoming from individuals who have lived through the sessions to now be able to reflect back over their experience to talk about it, especially in the sets of questions No. 6 and No. 7. Each one emphatically would do it again but might go about it differently. As a result, building upon Figure 2 from the previous pages, I postulate in *Figure 3* below that there can be *The Seven (7) Promises of Psychotherapy.* They are as follows:

1) The sooner you start, the more regularly you go, and the more often you come as you are to talk with someone objectively the quicker psychotherapy will work for you.

2) The more you expect only good to come from it, the more the good that will come from it.

3) The more you love yourself and others enough in order to improve your life, the more benefits you will discover.

4) If you take it seriously then it will seriously take care of you and you will get the most out of it.

5) The sooner you know it is "Okay" to be in therapy, the sooner you will accept the fact we all need advice at some time in our lives.

6) The quicker you embrace the purpose of being there, the quicker you will improve the way you think & feel because psychotherapy is healthy purging

7) The sooner you can trust the process, the sooner change will come in due time.

THE SEVEN-PROMISES OF PSYCHOTHERAPY

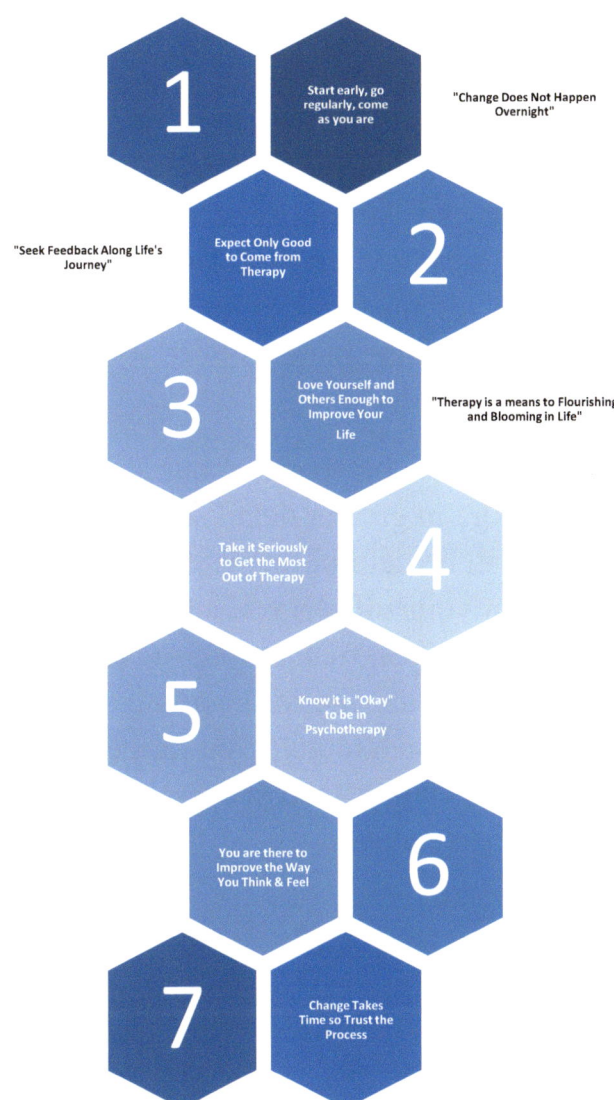

Figure 3

Whether or not we adhere to these particular rules of thumb, per se, is not as important as having some suggestions to go by from the patients' perspective. We each can go back through what the patients have said and possibly interpret other notions to draw from in relation to psychotherapy which is strongly encouraged here. In the meantime, these are the postulations advanced for now, points to take into consideration as we summarize what the patients have attempted to convey to us as the reader.

As we glean new perspective, our next chapter will explore in greater detail some further guidelines that will be helpful in approaching psychotherapy for yourself. As you integrate what the patients from these particular case studies have surmised, you too can use the forthcoming guidelines simply as such to help you further along this path of trying to understand psychotherapy from a patient's perspective.

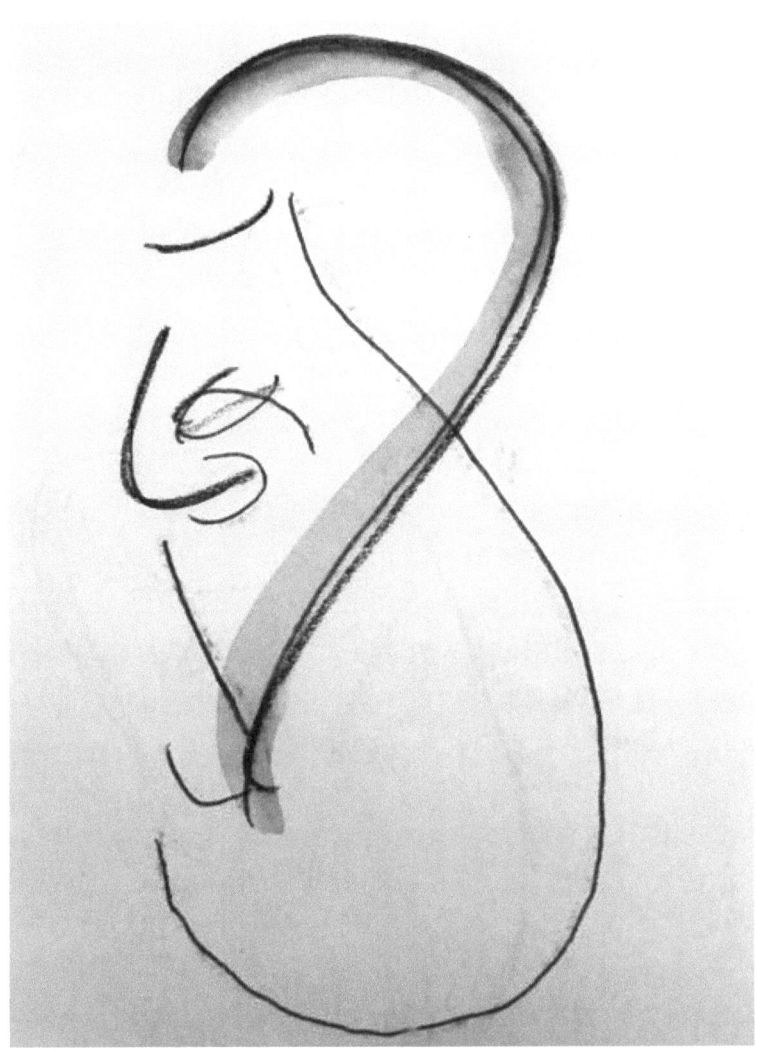

HALLMARK. Guidelines for the Game

Retitled watercolor on paper canvas with sketch tones
©2019 DR. PEIRSOL

CHAPTER 4
CLINICAL GUIDELINES OF THERAPY

Over the past 20 to 30 years of working with clients and patients alike, in either psychotherapy or life coaching, it has become apparent as a therapist, there are certain expectations patients have either directly or indirectly requested of me as their therapist. These expectations I consider to be guidelines toward helping me become a better psychotherapist. I have found that if I follow these guidelines for the most part, or the client's wishes when said and done, then the therapy tends to be more successful than not, and the patient benefits the most from the therapeutic experience more so altogether.

GUIDELINE NO. 1. When therapy starts, there are a lot of messages exchanged between the therapist and the client or patient. This exchange of information is the cornerstone of the psychotherapy. That is why it is critical that patient and therapist always understand each other. The therapist may readily try to make clear what they hear a patient say; but, many times patients tend to overlook or gloss over what is not clear that the therapist might have said. In the literature, it is reported that patients tend to compensate for the therapist's miscommunication in therapy. So, it is critical for you as the client to address this early on in treatment to improve the outcome of the therapy; however, patients tend to be reluctant to do so out of a feeling of deference for the therapist. It seems only natural however to address whatever comes up including the feelings that you need to protect the therapist. For example, let's say you just do not understand what the therapist is saying or there is a disconnect during the therapy experience. What we want to be able to say to the therapist is something like "Could you try running that by me again?" sort of scenario. The value of doing this will make sure what the therapist is trying to say is crystal clear for the client, just as much as it might seem clear to the therapist. Please understand that it is okay not understand what the therapist might be trying to say, but it is not okay to not let them know you do not understand what they are saying. It is not okay to carry on as if you understand when you don't. The reason for this is because much of therapy builds upon itself from one session to the next. What gets overlooked in one session will carry over into the next, slowing down or even curtailing the therapeutic experience altogether.

For example, therapists can miscue a patient's attempt to communicate a feeling or concern with or without words; so, as a patient, if at any time you feel as though you have not been heard correctly, whether you communicated well directly or not, or even indirectly (metacommunication),[x] and you still feel misunderstood, whether it is the result of you or the therapist miscuing, please be sure to *speak up.* **Guideline No. 1 is to speak up for yourself in therapy**. The more I have seen patients speak up for themselves in the therapy, the better the outcome of the therapy for all involved.

This need to speak up could be the result of you not liking the therapist's plan (questioning their approach), or wanting to understand but unsure how to grasp the therapist's "frame of reference" (p 431) and or finding simply the therapeutic environment does not suit you well. You simply are not comfortable for some reason. Or, you are just not sure how committed you are to the process and you have a "fear of examining threatening topics."[xi] Go ahead, get it out and speak up. The sooner you do, the better the therapeutic experience will be for you.

Other reasons to speak up according to Rennie (1994) include anxiety or fears surrounding your questioning the therapist, whether it is in censuring them to the point you might impact their self-confidence or sense of esteem as a professional. In other words, it is okay to second guess your therapist, the key though is to talk about it rather than keep it to yourself.

Other hesitancies include the struggle with "perceived expectations" you may have from the therapist and any assumed "indebtedness to the therapist" out of gratitude for how much the therapist has shown you their concern and support. Just because the therapist is the professional does not mean you have to conform on all points to be a stellar patient or client, to be the so-called "good client." It is okay to disagree with your therapist in other words. The sooner you state your perceived differences when they arise, the better the therapy and more positive the alliance with the therapist will be. This can appear counterintuitive at face value but in therapy it is more helpful as a patient to address any discrepancies especially if the therapist does not invite you to share any of your dissatisfactions. It is okay to offer your opinion; and remember, you will be all the better for it (p 431-36).

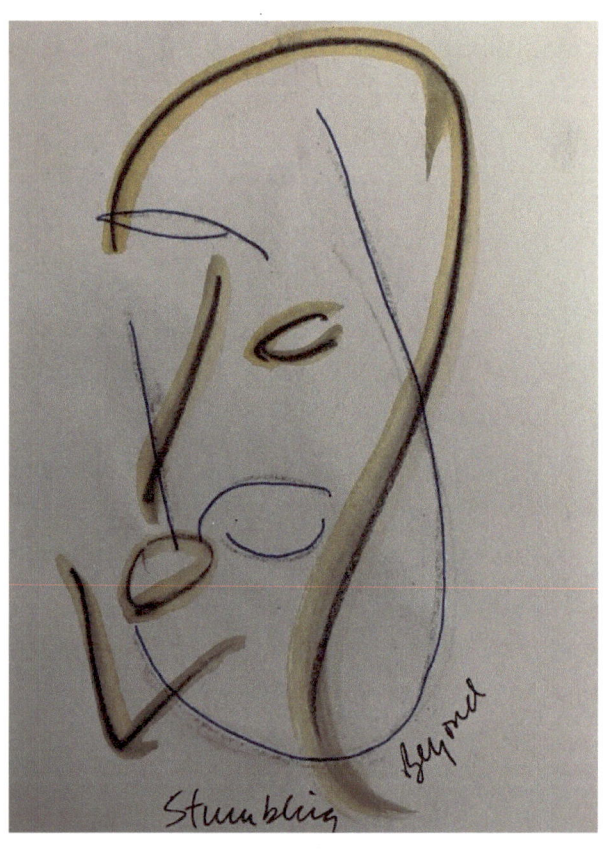

Watercolor on paper canvas with sketch tones
©2006 Dr. Peirsol

GUIDELINE NO. 2. When you get together with old friends, the idea is to get caught up on what's been happening in each other's lives. Or, when you use Facebook, the intention is to keep each other informed of what has been happening lately so everyone is up to speed on what is going on in your life. Similarly, we want to keep our therapist as informed as possible about what is happening as much outside of sessions as is what is happening during the session.

Levitt et al (2006) says there is a broad range of specifics that help regulate the therapeutic experience, ultimately though it is learning as a patient to always cultivate and maintain a relationship with your therapist that must "always" remain current; that is, never letting any unfinished business (or misperceptions) fester. This includes integrating what happens in session with what happens outside of session, addressing openly the question of how well you transition between the two within the alliance with the therapist. **Guideline No. 2 is to preserve an open and honest partnership with your therapist at all times.** The more I am made abreast of the comings and goings of patients, the better I am able to be there for my patients. And the better I am able to position myself in relation to their needs, then the better I am able to professionally help them reach their goals.

A lot happens in a session you will not necessarily be cognizant of until you experience a difference outside of a therapeutic session. Additionally, and naturally, a lot happens outside of session as well, especially things that maybe you are not so proud of and might be reluctant to share. Do not hold onto these secrets though, whether they occur from within the session when they arise during the session or from outside the session when they do occur as you are going on about your life. There is an old saying that a family is only as sick as the secrets they keep. This is true for us individually as well. Thus, the sorts of "Aha" experiences that do pop up as well as those sorts of "Oh no, I can't believe I did that!" experiences are the ones you want to bring up in session to process. This is not because you have to share but because the ultimate progression of therapy is a level of greater independence with the self-regulation of your own experiences outside of your relationship with your therapist. To do this, it first has to be fully regulated together before it can be transitioned back to you to better self-regulate. This takes time and to speed up the process means to address shifts, as well as experiences, as they arise to be sure you are reading the vicissitudes or variations in your life correctly, applying the new skills you are learning most efficiently along the way (pp 318-22).

In some schools of thought, the therapeutic relationship is *sine qua non* to effective psychotherapy- it is essential for it to work. Some theories are based solely on the effectiveness of the relationship while others utilize the alliance similarly as a vital element. For you as the patient, it basically is the means to an end with a little fluff in the middle. You have to make a good connection and at least understand each other, hopefully like one another to say the least. One way to accomplish this is to be straight forward, open and forthright at all times. Granted, it is hard to open up about things you might not be too proud of for example. The risk of feeling humiliated is sometimes enough to keep you from doing it, much less only then to be abashed for it by someone else. The best therapeutic alliance fosters unconditional regard and self-other-mutual acceptance. But, to do this you too have to participate. Be vulnerable at times, allow yourself the freedom to finally fully be just who you are with someone else, no-wholes-barred and no strings attached. Just let it rip. You will feel all the better for it and find the process of psychotherapy most refreshing as a result.

Many times, I will tell patients it is not the absence of pathology that makes them whole, but rather the level of awareness of it shared with another that lessens its toll. One less burden carried is the one that is finally shared. Many think "Why should I share it? It's past so what good will it do?" You will be amazed at what can happen when you open up with your therapist and share things maybe you have not told anyone. There is a level of inspiration derived from sharing that can make the difference in both the alliance with your therapist and the outcome of the therapy altogether. Again, both your motivation to work on the things that concern you and your focus on preserving this coalition with your therapist together are predictors of a better outcome. If you allow yourself to actively participate by 1) being accountable truthfully and honestly such as is suggested here, both introspectively as well as retrospectively and 2) remain willing "to change, explore, and experiment (with) curiosity (in an effort) to understand oneself" as well as 3) have "realistic expectations of the therapeutic outcome…(with) reasonable sacrifices" then you will know a fuller influence of the psychotherapy experience.[xii]

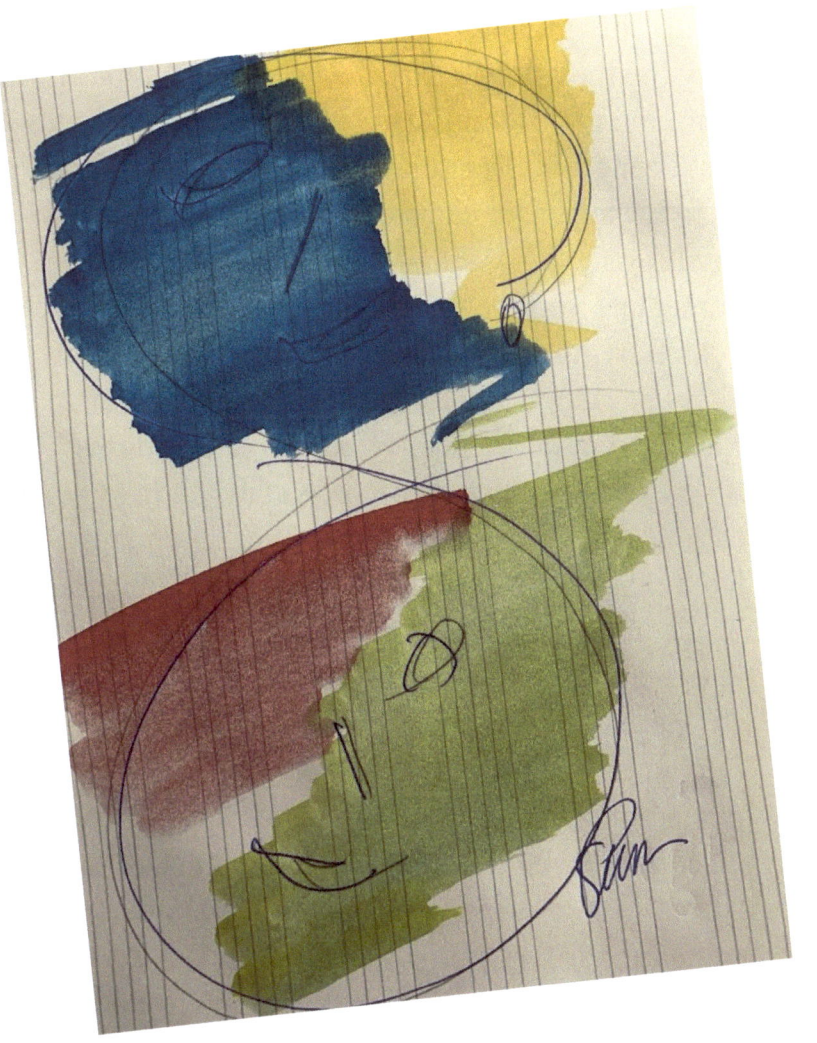

Untitled watercolor on paper canvas with sketch tones
©2019 Dr. Peirsol

GUIDELINE NO. 3. It takes time to open up fully in therapy but the more fully you open up, the more fully the therapeutic experience will be in return. It is not much different than being with one of your best friends, feeling rejuvenated just by being with them because you can freely be yourself without anything to worry about. Similarly, the more immediate you are in addressing your experiences in therapy, the more vibrant the experiences will likely be, less weighted down with thought and caution. Similarly, how effectively you address what arises in therapy just as you might in your natural life with a close friend, the lighter and livelier your life experiences will tend to be both inside and outside of therapy. **Guideline No. 3 is to openly trust your experience.** To do this is not always easy for all clients; however, the more freely one can go with the flow of the experience in therapy, the more quickly patients tend to adapt more effectively to their life circumstances.

You do not have to fully understand something to grasp it, even if it is by the tail you clasp it. In other words, hypothetically we do not have to be an expert in quantum physics to know that what generally goes up must come down. Nor do we have to fully understand our experiences on all their terms in order to live. The nature of psychotherapy is to help individual's to more fully embrace the fullness of their life experience in all its essence even if it is just a little bit at a time; otherwise, part of us can split off and get distorted or lost in the experience. This is when we find ourselves turning around, asking "What did I just miss?" or "What was that?" only to find we for some reason did not catch onto whatever it was that happened in the experience effectively enough.

For the most part, therapy in effect digs into our life experience to move us forward, to pick up that which was lost or missed in the past experience so we can move it frontward into our current life experience to live more integrated with our current experience- to more fully be in the present here and now. Once we comprehend this more readily, the more quickly we will find we can live our lives moving forward rather than tending backwards. This is why we must trust our experiences even though many times we question them. It will be our second guessing ourselves in our experiences or circumstances that we are unable to effectively understand the experience itself. Herein, psychotherapy can help "facilitate with safety the opening up of deep layers of the client's experience" realistically with the therapist in order to feel empowered to deal with it more self-respectably. This hastens the ability to enable greater relief from whatever distresses, "contributing to (an) ongoing personal development" ultimately beyond the therapeutic endeavor itself.[xiii]

If you find you are having difficulty with the idea of letting go in your life experiences, allowing your experience to take you wherever it may lead you, to trust it more openly, then it might be helpful to explore with your therapist skills surrounding *mindfulness.* Aside from the need to consider any meditative practices, the idea is not to alter the way you are but rather to simply adjust to how you are. Mindfulness is "a process of bringing a certain quality of attention to moment-by-moment experience(s)" in order to relieve maladjusted tendencies. One of the primary benefits of sharpening one's focus like this is to minimize the "emotional distress" that comes with life in general.[xiv] As a result, experiences do not always dictate outcomes but rather with sharpened skill, more conscious-acting decisions do. In my other books, *Psychotherapy-Let's Get Better* and *Bipolar Depression* there are sections devoted to the significance of this mindfulness skill especially with an emphasis upon its many health benefits as well. So, in effect, I cannot emphasize enough how important it is to work toward embracing your experience more openly especially in the therapeutic setting.

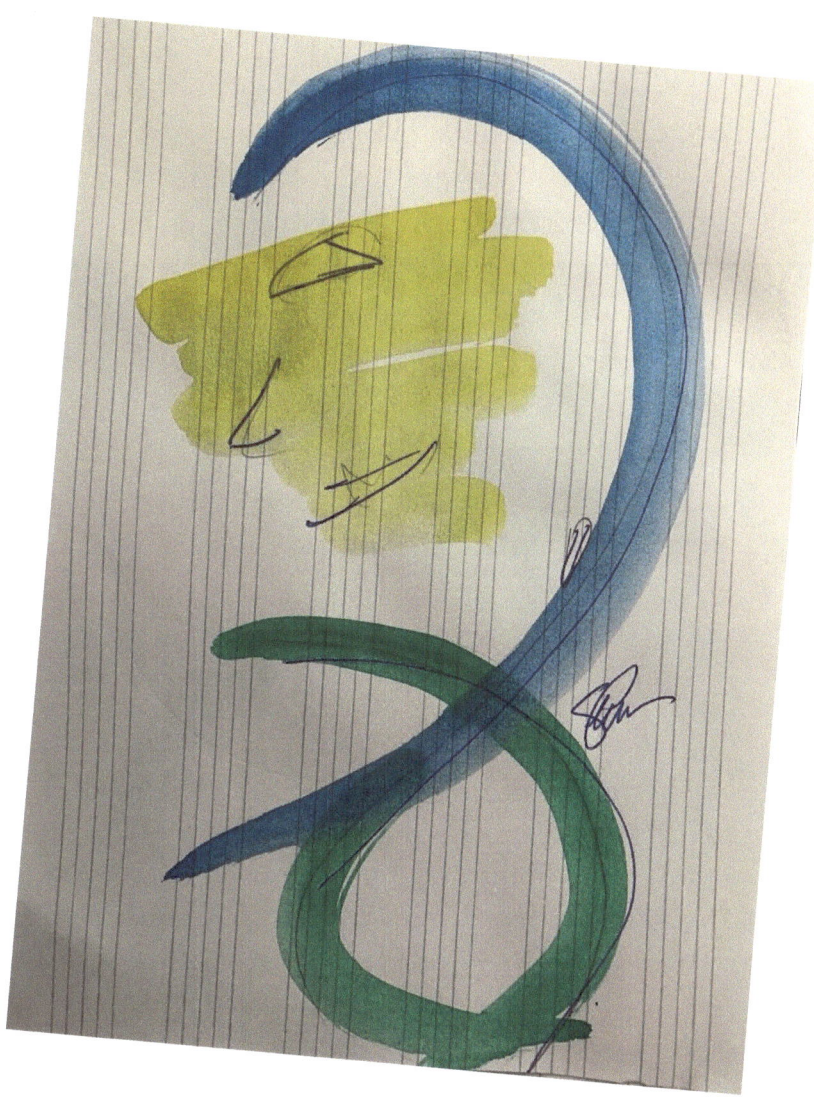

Untitled watercolor on paper canvas with sketch tones
©2019 Dr. Peirsol

GUIDELINE NO. 4. One of the big hang-ups with psychotherapy is the fact everyone tends to get labeled with a diagnosis. But for insurance claims this requirement might be obsolete. It is for billing purposes predominantly and prescription targeting clinically that these labels linger still as a problem for most; otherwise, there might be less of a tendency to use such tag names in the form of a diagnosis with patients. Yes, some people want to know what it is that bothers them, and this is understandable; however, the tendency is to gravitate toward the label and its implications rather than toward the symptoms that regulate it. All said, it is the symptoms we are addressing in psychotherapy anyway not necessarily the label. **Guideline No. 4 is to not obsess about your diagnosis.** A lot of time is spent on understanding what is going on, but do not let too much time be spent on the label of the diagnosis. Always try to remember a diagnosis is simply a new awareness about aspects of how we are and not an altered existence of who we are.

Keep in mind one of the other primary reasons for a diagnosis is for the clinician more than anything else. This is right. Clinicians staff together to discuss cases so they can help each other address patient needs, consider alternative techniques, various medications, etc., and one way to speed up this process is to identify a case by its diagnosis. "Patient X presents with…" this or that, and so on, more as a way to describe what is happening than to disregard in any way the identity of the person(s) involved. Unfortunately, however, patients (or clients), the person in therapy, etc., internalizes what the diagnosis is more as a representation of who they are rather than what they have. "I am depressed" verses "I have depression"; or, "I am bipolar" verses "I am dealing with a bipolar disorder." Better yet, in the adage of the AA *esprit de corps* "I am an alcoholic" verses "I am dealing with alcoholism" is what gets reinforced *en masse*.

Truer to color is the expression "I have cancer" verses saying, "I am breast cancer." Huh? Why then do we tend to be more self-deprecative when it comes to mental health labels? There are many reasons for sure, but probably the biggest one is because in our society mental illness is still considered taboo in many circles. As a result, all the labels that come with it are too. What I am suggesting instead is "to stop" letting it be offensive, scared, off limits, etc. *Just do not do it* instead of *just do it.* When it gets put that way, it almost feels counterintuitive; however, we need to work on maintaining a separation from what we have to deal with in a diagnosis verses who we are when it comes to being in psychotherapy. The sooner we can adjust to this the better off we will be.

To support this notion further, one of the difficulties in trying to get away from feeling stuck being labeled is the fact we feel like a part of us has been "displaced" and is now permanently different once we are branded. In some cases, the person feels like a "diseased entity." In addition, intrinsically we likewise begin to include others in our mind consciously especially when it comes to something negative. All at once, we find ourselves even more stuck and at the mercy of another's interpretation of us as the diagnosed one! We begin to feel alienated from others as a result of what seems like an "insult" whether this is true or not. The reason for this is we somehow start to think there is something wrong with us. Such alienation comes from what we interpret in our head rather than necessarily what is true about our body or mind. According to Knight et al (2003), Burston (1998)[xv] declares that to alienate actually implies a "'state or process whereby one becomes separated or estranged from one's original condition' (and) unfolds as something inconsistent with the notion of the evenness of being." Loneliness and isolation set in in other words. We feel a disconnect not only within ourselves because we do not understand, but we somehow believe we are subsequently alienated from others with the nagging belief we will simply not be understood by others either.

As a result, we start incessantly "monitoring" ourselves out of fear we will be found out without an opportunity to fully explain (p 3-14). In other words, we begin to concoct we are no longer on level playing field with others because of a diagnosis and we feel like we just got the short end of the stick. Something is now wrong with us and we are now damaged goods sort of thing. "I am not necessarily just 'me' without involving others around me; so, if I am dealing with this or that, (the diagnosis), then others too will have to deal with it (me) as well" and that all just doesn't look so good. Automatically we wonder what others will think and before long we lose ourselves in all these consternations.

Subsequently, these misinterpretations impact whether we choose to share what we are experiencing with someone else or not, a fundamental process referred to as *intersubjectivity* which is "foundational in situating the self in relation to others" (p 2). Our awareness of the "self" changes and we are then altered "through (our) awareness of (our) self-other relatedness." Martin Buber, the preeminent German philosopher from the early 1920's, put it this way- He said that the "self" was depicted as the "reciprocal recognition of the other." In other words, we all co-exist within and through each other by which the meaning of who we are or how one gets defined is established.[xvi] Harry Stack Sullivan, the seminal American psychiatrist, described this notion instead through his understanding of mental health itself. His conclusion was that mental health was not necessarily a state of being but rather a state of awareness in relation to others; more specifically, our level of awareness of our inter-relatedness with others defines our level of mental health.

Our unfortunate tendency however is that if we get a diagnosis then surely others will think differently of us, and so on, leaving us feeling uncertain about what will become of us as a result. When, in fact, *a diagnosis is simply a new awareness about aspects of how we are and not an altered existence of who we are.* Ultimately, just because one gets a diagnosis does not change who they are nor does it have to shape the relationships with and toward others unless we allow for it to. A diagnosis just describes by explanation, with much ambiguity too I might add, all the symptoms you may be experiencing, and does not define who you are. This depiction with a tag name does not define you but rather adds greater value to the substance of which you are made to get to the bottom of it.

In effect, a diagnosis becomes a matter of perspective based upon the experience of the tag name itself, the extent to which you allow yourself to share this "tag name" experience of yourself with others impacts both how you see yourself and your overall mental health. So, look at your diagnosis, if you get one, this tag name, as just one other part of the prism that makes you, you; that it does not define you, it just helps better describe you, just one other aspect of the experience of your life with whomever else you decide to share.

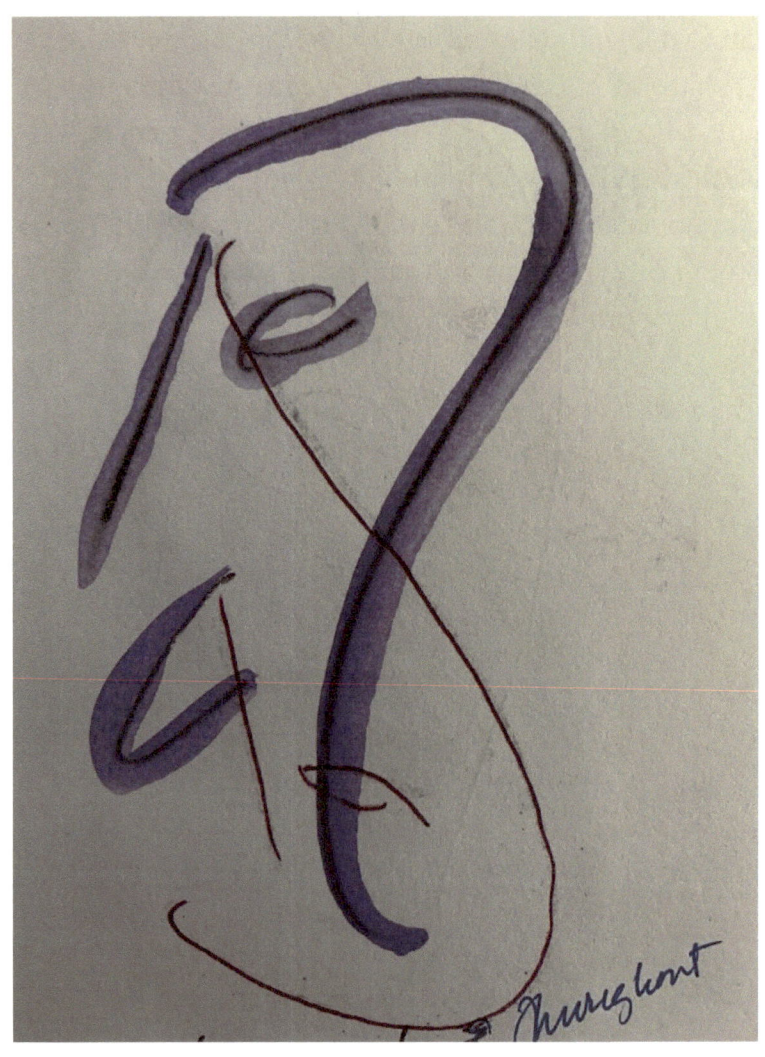

Over and above

Watercolor on paper canvas with sketch tones
©2019 Dr. Peirsol

GUIDELINE NO. 5. It is important to have a vision otherwise, according to Solomon, "people will perish." This applies to going into psychotherapy as well. When you start psychotherapy, it is not unusual to feel lost, unclear of "what's what" much less which direction to take because life might not be any longer as you once knew it. **Guideline No. 5 is to develop a vision for your current life circumstances that is concrete, clear and specific.** It is always important to maintain a clear goal while you in therapy, to know where you are where you are headed. This helps keep you grounded and more surefooted when there is a lot going on around you.

To be clear, this does not happen fast unless of course you already know what you want to address. Otherwise, it can take a long time to yield shape to this vision while in therapy. For example, let us say you discover you are dealing with some set-back that has you all bummed out. Your therapist runs some test that indicate a moderate depressive quality to it. As a result, you start on some anti-depressant medication to help. Before long you start feeling better even though the bummer of a thing that got you in there still has not panned out. So where to from here? You feel better but your problems still have not sorted themselves out. The dilemma is you came in to therapy to straighten out your messed-up plans, and they are crooked still, only to find you were depressed but now you feel better.

In other words, once in therapy, things can shift from this to that fairly quickly, altering frequently your best laid plans. To stay rock solid on your feet, typically your therapist will lay out a plan of action at the start you both need to agree upon- this way you work toward exactly what you want as a result of the psychotherapy experience. As you progress, be sure to address and redress the plan to keep it up to snuff with where you are in the process.

What is needed "is a framework for determining whether a therapist's interventions are well suited to a particular patient's problems and goals" (p 42) according to Silberschatz et al. (1989).[xvii] In other words, you drive the direction of the therapy with the assistance of the therapist's instrumentation along the way. Not the other way around. That is right, you initiate the direction of the therapy, remaining open to suggestions along the way, with a little nudge here and there considering any surprises such as the depression in this example along the way. Consequently, from the very beginning, try to state what it is you need and attempt with each session to have a goal even if it is simply to go in with an open mind, letting what happens to just happen *laisse faire*. You can even say "I don't know what I need, I just know I need something so please help." The more diligent you are about what you want the more you will get what you want out of it. It is not much different than most anything else you put your mind to. The more you put into it, the more you will get out of it.

Keep in mind psychotherapy considers most anything one could possibly talk about. This includes social issues, personal and spiritual ones as well. You can address emotional as well as mental matters as well as habits and feelings that either are helping you or hurting you. It can explore past issues or current ones, conscious or unconscious ones as well; what is helping you reach your goals and what is preventing you from attaining them; what insights you might need or what defenses might be blocking you from the source of your problems (p 41). You name it, within reason, and psychotherapy can address it.

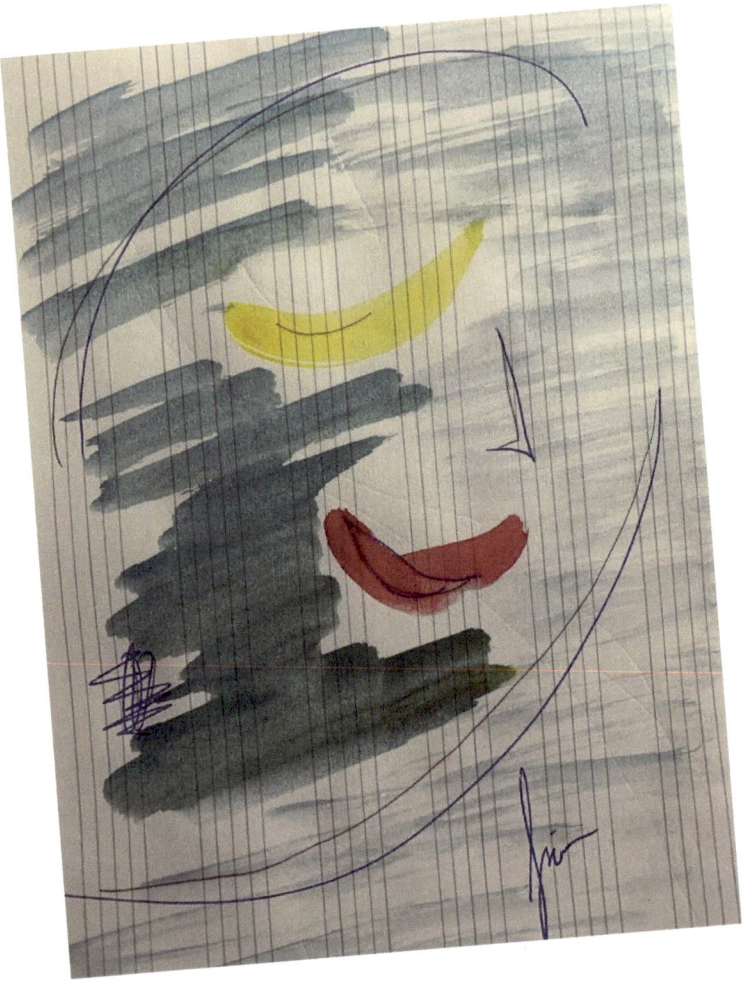

Untitled watercolor on paper canvas with sketch tones
©2019 Dr. Peirsol

GUIDELINE NO. 6. Usually by the time we realize we need someone who will listen, someone like a therapist who would tend to our concerns, our issues generally evolve to involve other people. Psychotherapy is never necessarily an isolated event. It generally involves someone or something other than just the patient themselves. **Guideline No. 6 is to include openly all those involved in your life as soon as possible.** There is strength in numbers is what I like to say sometimes, and the more you have rallying on your behalf the better.

Many theories consider all of the parties involved surrounding the so-called identified person who is in therapy; however, not all theoretical orientations openly address everyone involved. The key is to keep in mind the notion no one is necessarily an island unto themselves. Everybody functions in relation to someone else somehow, some way. In this way, be sure to bring whoever else might be involved in your life up in the therapy, whomever they might be, as soon as possible. This does not mean to bring everyone and their brother to the therapy. It just means to openly discuss your current relationships in the therapy.

One theorist, Carl Whitaker, a preeminent American psychiatrist, developed *Experiential Family Therapy*, proposing that togetherness and cohesion with others equates to growth because emotions form the ability for us to have attachments. He felt that emotions were the key communication factors in relationships and that they go hand-in-hand. Thus, for emotions to work properly, relationships have to be involved and vice versa. For example, if there is a self-esteem problem then there was likely a relationship problem somewhere in the mix and vice versa. He along with Virginia Satir, a distinguished psychotherapist, advanced further that relationship problems had a lot to do with emotional suppression and could be traced back to the family system of origin. As a result of such suppression, the *individuality* of the person was not respected and thus not properly developed.

This process of bringing all others involved to your therapeutic experience affords instead a therapeutic dialogue which allows for what Whitaker and Satir called *differentiation*, the means by which an individual can develop a healthier sense of autonomy emotionally. They advanced if there remained highly charged emotions currently for example, then the problem could be sketched back to previous generational complications that endure to the present.[xviii]

So, if there are emotional concerns then there are likely relationship concerns. Accordingly, be as open as possible about your relationships so any challenging ones can be identified and discussed to ensure your emotional individuality is fostered and fully reinforced. Harry Stack Sullivan, referred to earlier, also reinforced the importance of our interrelatedness here with others pertaining to our mental health; that his notion of mental health as a state of awareness verses a state of being focused upon others in relation to the self. So, the more quickly you can describe what is happening socially in your life, how well you are getting along with others, and your awareness of the impact of such relations, the more quickly you will find the effectiveness of the therapeutic experience.

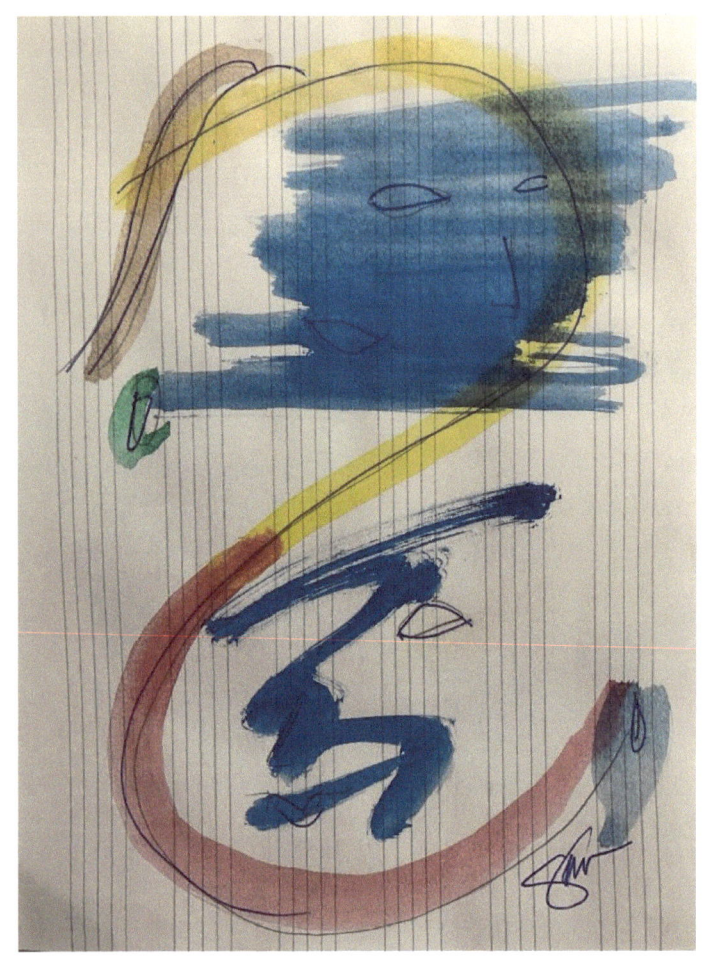

Untitled watercolor on paper canvas with sketch tones
©2019 Dr. Peirsol

GUIDELINE NO. 7. In psychotherapy, there is the experience between what has happened and what is yet to occur. This place is dwelling within a space where change takes place, sometimes referred to as *edge-sensing*, being on the edge of what is new, not yet formed, the edge of existence. In some schools of thought it is the place between what is referred to as trailing-edge verses leading-edge experience. **Guideline No. 7 is to focus your energies upon moving forward with life through psychotherapy.** Try to let your focus be on the possibilities and not the pathologies of psychotherapy, the future with all its opportunity rather than just the past and all its problems.

What lies behind is there to help propel you ahead in life rather than to drag you backwards with life. Yes, we need to look back to learn from what has transpired; however, we do not need to live in history in order to learn from it. Let us review the past to garnish what nuggets of truth or wisdom we can glean and move it forward to improve the decisions that lie ahead. Many times, clients will continue with life in the here and now but base it upon being stuck instead in old ways of thinking because of what they still feel from the past. The idea of moving forward means to not only be functioning well in the present but also feeling what is happening within the present.

Think of this way. I cannot function very well for example if I am hung over from the night before. Similarly, we cannot function well today if we are still feeling residuals from yesterday. Hence, this edge-sensing notion is one in which what has transpired in the past has been properly placed in the past and is in its place now to help with the present. The key here is what has passed helps now in the present.

Insights are important, altering one's way of thinking, and changing how one behaves or believes are all very important elements of psychotherapy; however, do not overlook the importance of dealing with what you directly feel in relation to what you concretely experience. As you change, remember to bring the feelings along with the change so all of your energy can be encapsulated rather than unnecessarily dispersed. By dispersed I mean misplaced or displaced verses being channeled or contained with one's experience. For example, one might get upset at work and end up kicking the dog when they get home. Those are displaced emotions. We want to have our cake and eat it too; that is, have the experience (good, bad or indifferent) and also feel whatever it is that comes with it rather than be cut-off from feeling whatever that experience brings.

The way to do this will become more self-evident in the therapy as you learn to listen more to your body and tap into what is referred to as "feeling knowledge" which stems from "sensory motor affective language" viscerally within the body. What generally happens is feelings surface implicitly in the therapeutic dialogue between patient and therapist, the therapist then in turn recognizing certain expressions the patient might not be cognizant of at the time. These feeling are acknowledged, addressed and processed with the patient until made more conscious. This process involves both intra and inter psychic connections explicitly that must be processed in the therapeutic relationship to enable the patient to move their emotions forward into their current experience. This then becomes habituated and the patient is able to do the same more comprehensively themselves without so much of the therapist's promptings. This externalization of emotions in turn becomes a new skill set empowering the patient more intrinsically to move forward in their life experience more intact emotionally. [xix]

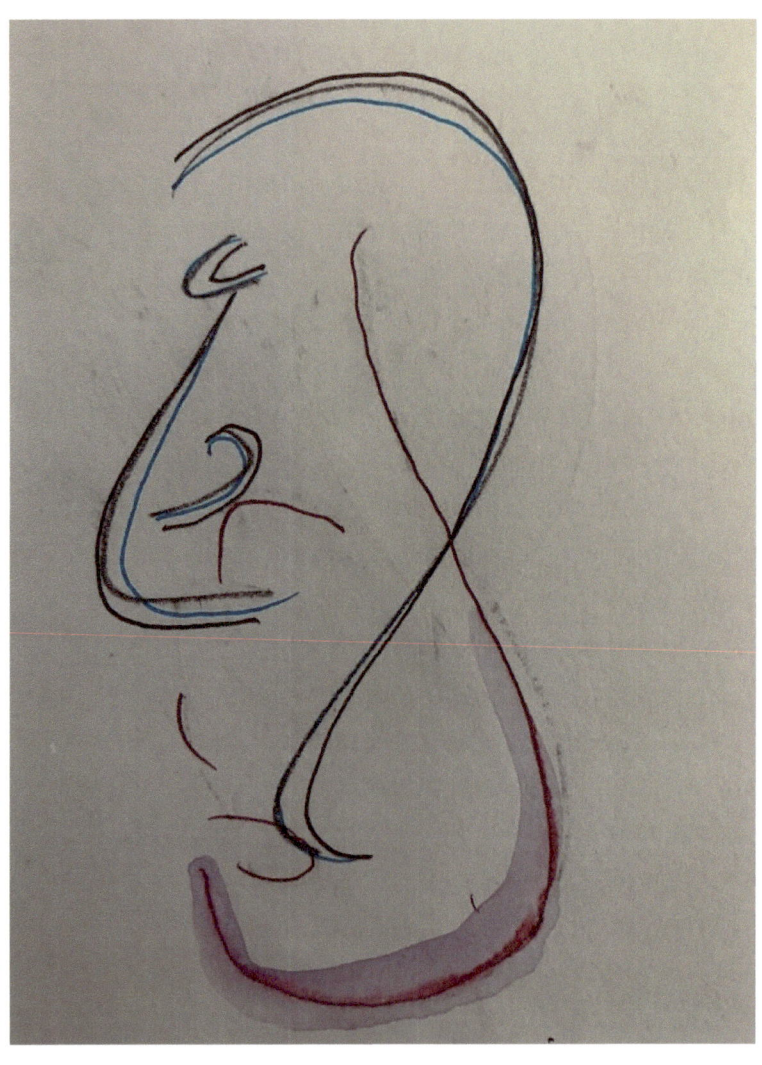

Untitled watercolor on paper canvas with sketch tones
©2006 Dr. Peirsol

GUIDELINE NO. 8. Wouldn't it be nice to be able to just tap an app on your smartphone and "Viola!" all your problems would just go "Poof!" in an instant. Or, if at the very least, once you tapped the app then all your feelings could instantly feel better. We do become accustomed to instant gratification, Amazon delivered in a box right at our doorstep, right on time every time. This is not the case when it comes to psychotherapy. **Guideline No. 8 is to be patient with your outcomes**. It is about accepting that change in psychotherapy takes its own sweet time. Just as it is said "When the therapist is ready then the patient will come"; so similarly, "When the patient is ready, the remedy will come." Part of the therapeutic work is in simply positioning yourself to receive new insight with greater awareness and it is by positioning yourself to be the best you can be right now that this insight with heightened awareness will come.

There are techniques that radically alter how one is feeling, especially when someone goes through hypnosis or some form of relaxation therapy; however, for the most part, psychotherapy has its own timeline when it comes to changing an individual's life. Wish it was different, and I could wave a magic wand to make it all better; but, the science has not advanced that far and most likely never will. It is still one day at a time approach, one session at a time, sometimes painstakingly slow in its process. However, the truth is in every session there is change. This is where I want you to focus: on the changes that do take place however slow, however small, at least focus upon what is changing.

Keep in mind the more significant one's problem, the greater the impact a change. Change might be more noticeable early on, what I call the "newness effect." Buy a new car and everything is better until the sweet new car smell wears off; that monthly payment starts to get old pretty fast. We do not want to look at psychotherapy in this way. Every session needs to be new. Yes, the newness effect will take place and you will probably be feeling somewhat better after your first few sessions; however, deep characterological changes take time and we have to be able to break change down into small compartments. Characterological factors deeply engrained warrant more time and effort to change however specific areas of change can be monitored and evaluated weekly.

For example, let us assume we are dealing with depression. This is not as simple as diagnosis, talk, and "Boom!" you are done. There are ways of thinking, feeling and acting that contribute to depressive tendencies, all which warrant examination. So, take one aspect at a time. Look at how you view your life and see if there is anything different about it now that you have been talking about it? Have you noticed you are less fastidious about all the details and maybe a little more foot loose and fancy free than you used to be possibly? Or, are you better able to overlook the small things that used to get you down and begin to view instead the big picture from a brighter perspective? Do these shifts happen without you thinking about it, start to occur more naturally just as a byproduct of you being you?

When you look at this Guideline, do not forget that you are hardwired to get well. That is right. The hardwiring is such that it works toward getting better in the same way our body heals itself. Similarly, our psyche seeks to do the same. It just might take a little longer. For example, not too long ago I cut my left hand on some glass. Had to get about 20-stitches. It looked gnarly at first, cut and bruised, all stitched with scars here and there. Bloody and dark. Gradually however it became blemish free. It was amazing, as if nothing ever happened. Now I can type away on my keyboard, carry things, move my had freely; and, to look at my hand, you would never know I had some 20-stitches in it just months ago. Similarly, our psyche might be wounded, hypothetically getting some metaphorical 20-stitches; however, it will not heal like the hand, returning to its original form. Instead the psyche will mend where it can and compensate where it cannot, forming instead a makeshift comparison to what used to exist before the injury, always similar to how it used to be but never the same. Always better but just not alike. And, it will be up to us to learn how to re-orchestrate what is new into what works for us, slowly but surely.

The bottom line is that although psychotherapy may take its sweet time to inject change, what is happening all the while is our "psychosocial resilience (is orchestrating our own) human psychological development (in a) highly buffered and self-righting'' way according to Masten, Best, and Garmazy (1990)[xx] emphasized by Bozart (2000).[xxi] In other words, our psyche is righting itself much like a hand-held compass as you turn side to side, and the pointer flickers to the right and then to the left, correcting itself to provide the exact direction due. The pointer keeps moving until you are still, and it gives you the exact waypoint once it has settled. Similarly, as our life gets tossed to the right and then to the left at times, our psyche keeps adjusting much like the compass's pointer until it finally reaches its centering point and settles back into its regulating waypoint(s).

For those of you that might have sailed can truly relate to this analogy. This interesting comparison can be extended similarly because on certain navigating devices, one can pre-chart the waypoints, the longitude and latitude destination(s) from the chart. In this way, once the waypoints are input, you simply can set to sail and navigate instead with the predestined waypoints on the device verses constantly looking at the chart to adjust your heading. Instead, the navigation equipment has the waypoints logged in for you to just adjust your sails and reutter accordingly. This provides for a much more leisurely sail.

The first time I programmed a device like this, my brother and I were sailing back from the Abaco Islands to the east coast of Florida, targeting the inlet of Daytona Beach, just north of New Smyrna Beach inlet where we grew up surfing as kids. I pre-programmed all the necessary waypoints on this new device and "Viola!" we hit our destination right on. The saving grace was we hit a dead-calm while sailing back and it was these preprogrammed waypoints that kept us headed in the right direction the whole time. Being at sea, much like with life, it too takes its own sweet time as well. Once at sail, the saying "I'll get there when I get there" is so true. Even though we were days behind due to this dead-calm, we still hit all our waypoints. In fact, we hit them so well, our family could see us at sail from the New Smyrna Beach shoreline, and we could see them as well as we sailed in along the coast just south of the inlet.

Likewise, although we cannot exactly pre-program our psyche, we can however make the necessary adjustments therapeutically while it pre-programs itself. That is one of the finer tuned benefits of psychotherapy; that it can tap into a prewired system, our psyche, to help navigate us through life, irrespective of what might lie out at sea.

In summary, I have presented *8-Psychotherapy Guidelines* that will help enhance your therapy experience, guidelines that over the years patients have practice and found successful in their therapy. These guidelines are simply suggestions and they are presented here for your review in *Figure 4* below.

EIGHT-PSYCHOTHERAPY GUIDELINES

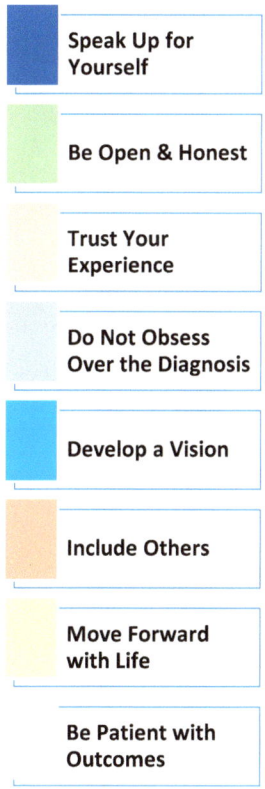

Speak Up for Yourself

Be Open & Honest

Trust Your Experience

Do Not Obsess Over the Diagnosis

Develop a Vision

Include Others

Move Forward with Life

Be Patient with Outcomes

Figure 4

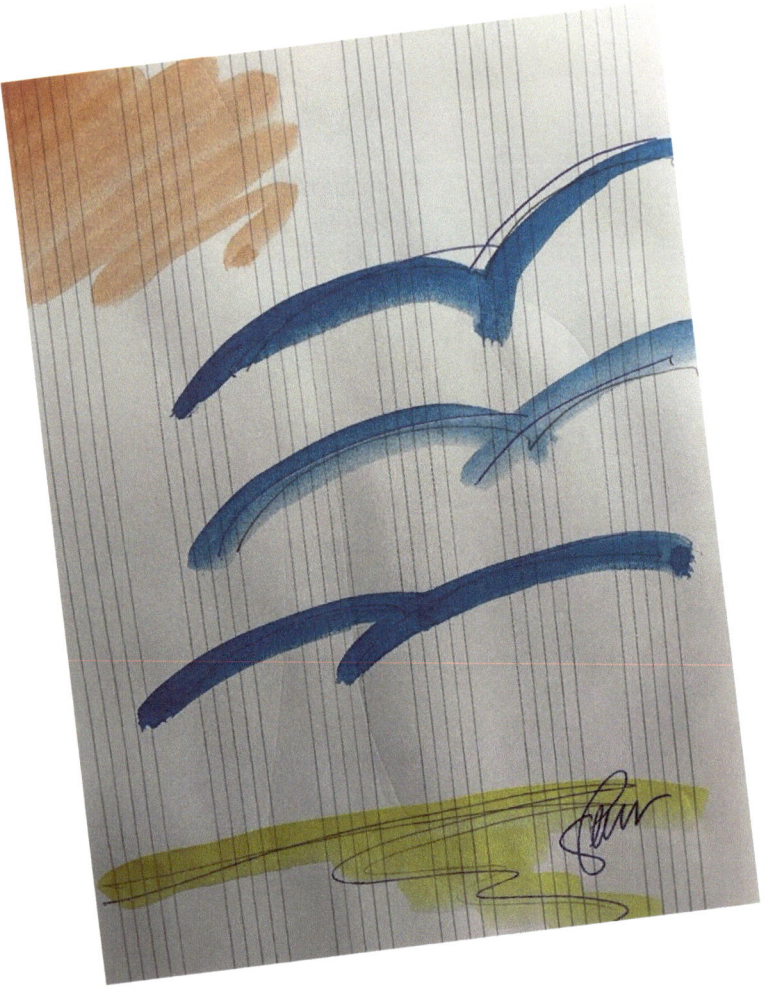

Take Flight

Watercolor on paper canvas with sketch tones

©2019 Dr. Peirsol

SUMMARY

The ideas gained from this book, *Psychotherapy from the Patient's Perspective*, are as empowering as the patients themselves who shared their stories; that what they have had to offer likewise empowers you as the reader to get the most out of therapy for yourself.

This idea of going to psychotherapy itself varies by each person's own personal experience but emphatically the case has been made that it is better to go to psychotherapy rather letting any reluctancy to get the best of you. Everyone recommended therapy as a result of their experience. No one shot it down. Additionally, the approach should be one of high expectancy, to anticipate good things to come from the psychotherapy. In other words, you can expect it to be a good experience for you, not a bad one. The ability to connect strongly with your therapist especially in those first few sessions, will allow for reinforcement in helping you make whatever decisions you are seeking to make in improving the quality of your life. Ultimately, the intention should be to go for it, and to remain open to whatever might occur along the way because it will be good.

Once the momentum gets started, we highlighted *10-Therapist Factors* supported in the literature to improve one's psychotherapy experience. It is nice to know that the experience of therapy will build upon the alliance of the therapeutic relationship; that you should anticipate there will be more positive interactions with your therapist than negative ones; that you will be able to rely upon the social support of your therapist and to remain engaged at all times with your therapist, eliciting more emotional responses along the way from your therapist that will be helpful to you along the way. In addition, it is nice to know that you will be able to rely upon the therapist's personal attributes, their personalness, their ability to tolerate closeness and to reduce anxiety in the alliance you will be sharing together while they discover with you better ways to relate with you more effectively. In effect, the psychotherapy will instill ongoing hope with curiosity that has the results you are looking for.

We also discovered that it will be important to remain open to continued life altering experiences in the therapy; that the impact of therapy will be beyond what you could imagine or ever fully anticipate, that you will be gaining on opportunities to improve the quality of your life the more quickly you start going and that what you have to learn will benefit you sooner than later in life the sooner you decide to go.

The case has also been made for *12-Takeaways from Psychotherapy* to offer others who intend to attend. As far as psychotherapy goes, one needs to go early and often, that it is a win-win proposition and you do not have to be strong to do it. We discovered it will change things for the better and help you take control of your life in ways you might not have anticipated. In addition, we explored the *Four (4) Rules of Thumb for Psychotherapy*: Start early, expect only good, take it seriously, and love yourself in the process. If you do these four tasks, then there is a much larger chance you will be able to get the most out of the process and see benefits sooner than later. The idea is to come as you are by going regularly, to expect only good to come from it, to take it seriously to get the most out of it, and to love yourself and others enough to improve your life through psychotherapy.

Additionally, we discovered *The Seven Promise of Psychotherapy*. We reinforced the importance of avoiding the stigma associated with going to psychotherapy, that it is "A-Okay to be in therapy" because it will improve the quality of your life. We also realized that change takes time but the time it takes is worth it in psychotherapy because what may have happened in the past will no longer define you as you move your life forward.

In conclusion, we established *8-Clinical Guidelines* for you to get the most out of psychotherapy. So, it is important to remember to succeed in therapy you want to speak up when you start, remain open to the process as you go along, welcome increased awareness to both he problems (diagnosis) that may arise as well as the success that is inevitable. Be sure and be visionary in the process while you include those important to you as you move it forward; and, remain patient with the process because it will all come together in its own specified time as you allow psychotherapy to work its work for you in your life.

ACKNOWLEDGMENTS

Acknowledgements go out to the patients courageous enough to tell their story, to talk about their experience in their own words, willing to open up and share so others too can benefit from their knowledge of making the most of psychotherapy.

Many thanks to all the patients that participated in creating this book. A special acknowledgement to one patient especially who passed away during the writing of this book. The book is dedicated in memory of them and in support of their family. "May those who read this book be as inspirational as you were in life, my friend, to all those who had the privilege of knowing you." Not enough words can be written to express the gratitude for this person's heart and soul that they poured out in psychotherapy, applying all the nuts and bolts that this book has to offer to the best of their ability, for reaping the full benefits of psychotherapy as they did so now others too can get the most of psychotherapy as well.

References

[i] Hersoug, A. G., Høglend, P., Monsen, J. T., & Havik, O. E. (2001). Quality of working alliance in psychotherapy: therapist variables and patient/therapist similarity as predictors. *The Journal of psychotherapy practice and research*, *10*(4), 205–216. Found on the internet May 16, 2019 at https://www.ncbi.nlm.nih.gov/pmc/articles/PMC3330657/

[ii] Lingiardi, V, Muzi, L, Tanzilli, A, Carone, N. Do therapists' subjective variables impact on psychodynamic psychotherapy outcomes? A systematic literature review. *Clin Psychol Psychother*. 2018; 25: 85– 101. Found on the internet May 16, 2019 at https://doi.org/10.1002/cpp.2131

[iii] Nissen-Lie, H. A., Havik, O. E., Høglend, P. A., Rønnestad, M. H., and Monsen, J. T. (2015) Patient and Therapist Perspectives on Alliance Development: Therapists' Practice Experiences as Predictors. *Clin. Psychol. Psychother.*, 22: 317– 327. Found on the internet May 16, 2019 at doi: 10.1002/cpp.1891.

[iv] Ulberg, R. , Amlo, S. , Hersoug, A. G., Dahl, H. J. and Høglend, P. (2014), The Effects of the Therapist's Disengaged Feelings on the In-Session Process in Psychodynamic Psychotherapy. J. Clin. Psychol.,

70: 440-451. Found on the internet May 16, 2019 at doi:10.1002/jclp.22088

[v] Colli, Antonello & Ferri, Martina (2015). Patient personality and therapist countertransference *Current Opinion in Psychiatry*: Volume 28 Issue 1 p 46–56 Found on the internet May 16, 2019 at doi: 10.1097/YCO.0000000000000119

[vi] Ackerman, Steven J. & Hilsenroth, Mark J. (2003) A review of therapist characteristics and techniques positively impacting the therapeutic alliance, *Clinical Psychology Review,* Volume 23, Issue 1, Pages 1-33. Found on the internet May 16, 2019 at ISSN 0272-7358, https://doi.org/10.1016/S0272-7358(02)00146-0

[vii] Black, S., Hardy, G., Turpin, G. and Parry, G. (2005), Self-reported attachment styles and therapeutic orientation of therapists and their relationship with reported general alliance quality and problems in therapy. *Psychology and Psychotherapy: Theory, Research and Practice*, 78: 363-377. Found on the internet May 16, 2019 at doi:10.1348/147608305X43784

[viii] Degnan, A., Seymour-Hyde, A., Harris, A., and Berry, K. (2016) The Role of Therapist Attachment in Alliance and Outcome: A Systematic Literature Review. *Clin. Psychol. Psychother.*, 23: 47– 65. Found on the internet May 16, 2019 at doi: 10.1002/cpp.1937.

[ix] Schattner, E., Tishby, O., and Wiseman, H. (2017) Relational Patterns and the Development of the Alliance: A Systematic Comparison of two

Cases. *Clin. Psychol. Psychother.*, 24: 555– 568.
Found on the internet May 16, 2019 at
doi: 10.1002/cpp.2019.

[x] Rennie, David L. (1994). *Clients' deference in psychotherapy.* Journal of Counseling Psychology, Vol 41 (4) 427-37.

[xi] Levitt, Heidi, Butler, Mike, & Hill, Travis. (2006). *What clients find helpful in psychotherapy: Developing principles for facilitating moment-by-moment change.* Journal of Counseling Psychology, Vol 53 (3) 314-24.

[xii] Rumpold, Gerhard, Doering, Stephan, Smrekar, Ulrike, Schubert, Christian, Koza, Ruth, Schatz, Dieter S., Bertl-Schuessler, Annemarie, Janecke, Nicola, Lampe, Astrid & Schuessler, Gerhard. (2005). *Changes in motivation and the therapeutic alliance during a pretherapy diagnostic and motivation-enhancing phase among psychotherapy outpatients.* Psychotherapy Research, January 15(1-2): 117-27. Found on the internet March 14, 2019 at https://www.researchgate.net/profile/Stephan_Doering2/publication/221676833_Changes_in_motivation_and_the_therapeutic_alliance_during_a_pretherapy_diagnostic_and_motivation-enhancing_phase_among_psychotherapy_outpatients/links/55e475f308aede0b573570be.pdf

[xiii] Sherwood, Trish. (2001). *Client experience in psychotherapy: What heals and what harms?* The Indo-Pacific Journal of Phenomenology Vol 1 (Ed 2) September (1-16). Found online March 12,

2019 at file:///C:/Users/drpei/Downloads/65705-131059-1-PB%20(1).pdf

[xiv] Bishop, Scott R., Lau, Mark, Shapiro, Shauna, Carlson, Linda, Anderson, Nicole D., Carmody, James, Segal, Zindel V., Abbey, Susan, Speca, Michael, Velting, Drew & Devins, Gerald. (2004). *Mindfulness: A proposed operational definition.* Clinical Psychology: Science and Practice, Autumn 11(3) Health Module, p 230-241. Found March 15, 2019 on internet at https://s3.amazonaws.com/academia.edu.documents/38930481/mindfulness-_a_proposed_operational_definition.pdf?AWSAccessKeyId=AKIAIWOWYYGZ2Y53UL3A&Expires=1552654262&Signature=O1cWCXAgtXY90ghZ2Q%2B%2FQbq4wUg%3D&response-content-disposition=inline%3B%20filename%3DMindfulness-_a_proposed_operational_defi.pdf

[xv] Burston, D. (1998). *Laing and Heidegger on alienation.* Journal of Humanistic Psychology, 38, 80- 93.

[xvi] Knight, Zelda G & Bradfield, Bruce C (2003) *The Experience of Being Diagnosed with a Psychiatric Disorder: Living the Label,* Indo-Pacific Journal of Phenomenology, 3:1, 1-20, DOI: 10.1080/20797222.2003.11433882. Found on the internet March 12, 2019 at https://www.tandfonline.com/doi/pdf/10.1080/20797222.2003.11433882

[xvii] Silberschatz, George, Curtic, John T., & Nathans, Shelley. (1989). *Using the patient's plan to*

assess progress in psychotherapy. Psychotherapy Vol 26 (1) Spring. Found on the internet March 13, 2019 at
https://www.researchgate.net/profile/George_Silber schatz/publication/232545712_Using_the_patient% 27s_plan_to_assess_progress_in_psychotherapy/lin ks/566087b108aebae678aa1e94/Using-the-patients-plan-to-assess-progress-in-psychotherapy.pdf

[xviii] Hutchinson, Linton. (2019). NationalCounselingExam.com. Found on the internet December 17, 2018 at
https://nationalcounselingexam.com/dashboard

[xix] Glanzer, David & Early, Annmarie. (2012). The role of edge-sensing in experiential psychotherapy. *American Journal of Psychotherapy* 66(4) p 391. Found on the internet April 15, 2019 at
https://doi.org/10.1176/appi.psychotherapy.2012.66. 4.391

[xx] Masten, A. S., Best, K. M., & Garmazy, N. (1990). Resilience and development: Contribution from the study of children who overcome adversity. *Development and Psychopathology*, 2, 425–444.

[xxi] Bohart, Arthur (2000). The client is the most important common factor: Client's self-healing capacities and psychotherapy. *Journal of Psychotherapy Integration.* 10(2) pp 133-34.

www.ingramcontent.com/pod-product-compliance
Lightning Source LLC
Chambersburg PA
CBHW041059180526
45172CB00001B/25